WHAT NURSES KNOW...
H I V / A I D S

WHAT NURSES KNOW...

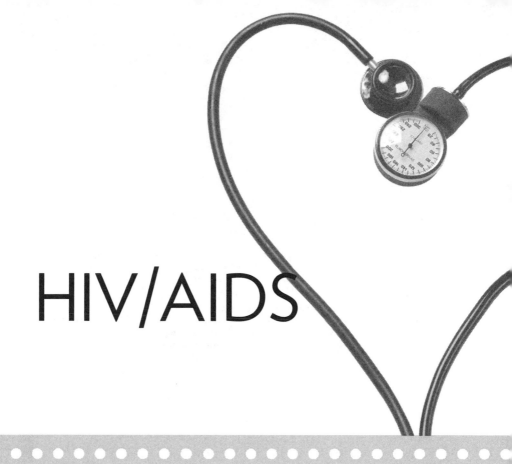

HIV/AIDS

Rose Farnan, RN, BSN, ACRN
Maithe Enriquez, RN, ANP-BC, PhD

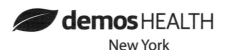

demos HEALTH

New York

ISBN: 978-1-936303-19-9
E-ISBN: 978-1-617050-84-8
Visit our web site at www.demoshealth.com

Acquisitions Editor: Noreen Henson
Compositor: Newgen

Medical information provided by Demos Health, in the absence of a visit with a health care professional, must be considered as an educational service only. This book is not designed to replace a physician's independent judgment about the appropriateness or risks of a procedure or therapy for a given patient. Our purpose is to provide you with information that will help you make your own health care decisions.

The information and opinions provided here are believed to be accurate and sound, based on the best judgment available to the authors, editors, and publisher, but readers who fail to consult appropriate health authorities assume the risk of injuries. The publisher is not responsible for errors or omissions. The editors and publisher welcome any reader to report to the publisher any discrepancies or inaccuracies noticed.

Library of Congress Cataloging-in-Publication Data

CIP data is available from the Library of Congress

Printed in the United States of America by Hamilton Printing
12 13 14 15 / 5 4 3 2

Rose Farnan, RN, BSN, ACRN, has been providing care to persons living with HIV for over 20 years in the Infectious Disease Clinic at Truman Medical Center, Hospital Hill in Kansas City. In her current role as infectious disease program manager, she manages several HIV-related programs, provides education to the community, and partners with many community organizations to improve care and reduce the stigma for people living with HIV.

Maithe Enriquez, RN, PhD, ANP-BC, is an advanced practice nurse who has specialized in HIV care for the past 18 years. In 2004, she completed a postdoctoral research fellowship at the University of North Carolina at Chapel Hill, focusing on the development of practical interventions to enhance health outcomes for individuals living with HIV and other chronic illnesses. She is an associate professor of nursing and assistant clinical professor of medicine at the University of Missouri–Kansas City. She has an active clinical practice in the Infectious Diseases Clinic at Truman Medical Center, Hospital Hill in Kansas City. Her research endeavors center on reducing health disparities and enhancing health outcomes for at-risk populations.

WHAT NURSES KNOW...

Nurses hold a critical role in modern healthcare that goes beyond their day-to-day duties. They share more information with patients than any other provider group, and are alongside patients twenty-four hours a day, seven days a week, offering understanding of complex health issues, holistic approaches to ailments, and advice for the patient that extends to the family. Nurses themselves are a powerful tool in the healing process.

What Nurses Know gives down-to-earth information, addresses consumers as equal partners in their care, and explains clearly what readers need to know and want to know to understand their condition and move forward with their lives.

I never thought in 1991 that 20 years later I'd still be working as a nurse in HIV care. I have learned so much from the many men and women I have met over the years, all living with HIV and allowing me to share a small part of their lives. Their dignity and courage when facing some of the most difficult of life's challenges have inspired me and, in turn, challenged me to continue in this field. I have also been guided and mentored by many phenomenal nurses, doctors, and case managers all dedicated to caring for people living with HIV, including my coauthor Maithe Enriquez. This book is dedicated to them and to all people living with HIV and the people who care for them, their families, friends, and healthcare workers.

—Rose Farnan

I dedicate this book to three very important people in my HIV career. First, Mr. Karl Cropsey, a friend and later a patient, who made me promise that I would always take care of myself first, so I'd have the energy to help my patients win their battle against HIV. Karl, a great man, lost his battle with HIV in 1995. Second, Dr. David McKinsey, an infectious diseases physician who has dedicated a significant portion of his career to bringing experimental and state-of-the-art HIV treatment to the people of our community. And finally, to my coauthor Ms. Rose Farnan, an outstanding role model for what nursing is all about.

—Maithe Enriquez

Contents

Foreword

As the fourth decade of living with HIV/AIDS begins, there has been a continuing shift in focus. The trajectory of infection and the needs of those affected have shifted as well. Nurses continue to be in the forefront of this change as they have been since the beginning of the epidemic. Yet too many people are newly acquiring HIV infection in this country and in other parts of the world. Worldwide, approximately 2.5 million persons become HIV infected each year and about 33 million persons are currently living with HIV infection. Although the appropriate antiretroviral therapy is available for direct treatment that can also reduce transmission chances, economic choices and allocations and sociopolitical agendas continue to influence treatment access and availability.

This entry in the series *What Nurses Know...* is both timely and important. Persons with HIV infection are living longer and longer. It has become incumbent upon them, along with their partners, their friends, and their families (however defined), to acquire knowledge and make decisions about short- and long-term treatment and care along with their healthcare providers. But how is such knowledge acquired? One important way is through the expertise of nursing professionals who have an understanding of HIV/AIDS and its related issues, and who are knowledgeable in what information to transmit to affected persons and the best ways in which to accomplish that.

Rose Farnan and Maithe Enriquez together have a greater number of years of clinical expertise in the HIV field than the years since HIV/AIDS has been recognized. They understand what affected persons need to know as well as the varying holistic and cultural dimensions to that knowledge through their own professional practices among the population affected by HIV/AIDS in the greater Kansas City area. Their expertise has led them to acquiring and sharing such knowledge among nurses and other healthcare practitioners on the national scene as well.

The first chapter delineates the important basics of what HIV and AIDS are in language that is clear and easy to understand. Following that is a chapter on what to do and what happens once the person knows that they have acquired HIV. Various potential additional resources are provided. Other vital issues that are covered include: managing HIV infection; forming healthy life habits and changing lifestyle; what medications are available and how to use them, and just as importantly, how to "stay with" them; infections related to HIV; mental health; substance abuse; men's and women's health; legal issues; sexuality and love life; having a family; and importantly, how to help a loved one with HIV/AIDS.

Each chapter begins with a short anecdote written by an HIV-affected person. Each chapter also has special highlighted sections of particularly helpful information called "What Nurses Know...." The sections are also chock-full of useful tips such as multiple practical ways to soothe a sore mouth when the mouth is infected or irritated. Further, there is a glossary of terms used, additional resources, and fact sheets.

Every person who faces the challenge of living with HIV infection or assisting a friend or loved one with HIV will benefit from this "must have" book written from the perspective of these two advanced practice nursing experts who are "out there" practicing in the real world.

Felissa R. Lashley, RN, PhD

Dean Emeritus and Professor Emeritus

School of Nursing

Southern Illinois University at Edwardsville

and

Past Dean and Professor Emeritus

College of Nursing

Rutgers, the State University of New Jersey

Acknowledgments

I thank two physicians whose dedication to patient care has inspired me to do more than I ever would have: Larry Dall, MD, the former chief of Infectious Diseases at Truman Medical Center, who never said "no" to any of my ideas and encouraged me to do all I could to help our patients. And David Bamberger, MD, the current chief of Infectious Diseases, whose commitment to excellence pushes me to exceed my limits. I thank my family, especially my parents, who not only supported my decision to care for people living with HIV, but even 20 years ago took every opportunity to express their pride in my decision. And, like Maithe, I will never be able to fully express my appreciation to the many men and women living with HIV who through the years have opened my eyes to social injustice and taught me how to truly be a nurse. They were, and continue to be, my heroes.

Rose Farnan

I thank all the individuals with HIV disease that I have had the privilege of taking care of over the past 18 years. I thank them for letting me be a part of their lives. I have learned most of what I know about HIV disease from them. They have taught me what it takes to fight the battle against HIV and win! I also thank my colleagues at Truman Medical Center, Infectious Diseases Associates, Guadalupe Center, and the University of Missouri-Kansas City for their support of our patients and our HIV research endeavors. Finally, I thank my husband, daughter, nieces and nephews, parents, siblings and siblings-in-law, grandmother, aunts, uncles, and cousins (affectionately known as "La Familia") for their support and love.

Maithe Enriquez

WHAT NURSES KNOW . . .

HIV / AIDS

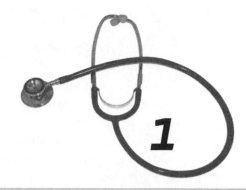

What Is HIV?
What Is AIDS?

Five years ago, my husband and I found out that I was pregnant. We were so happy and excited. My husband took off from work to go to my first prenatal appointment. That first appointment was a blur. There were all kinds of forms to fill out, and they drew blood for a lot of tests. They asked my husband and me all kinds of questions about our health. Everything seemed to go ok. Then I received a call 2 weeks later. The nurse asked if I could come back in for the doctor to go over some lab tests with me. My husband couldn't get off work, so I went alone. I was so scared something was wrong with the baby. I never expected to be told I had HIV. I think I went into shock. I was numb. I didn't believe that the lab tests were right. I called and made an appointment at a free health clinic and went and got tested again. The results were the same. I had..... I have HIV.... I'm HIV positive. ALICIA, AGE 27

You, or someone you know, may have just been told you have HIV. Denial is a very common response when you hear that you have a disease like HIV—a disease that could impact your health for a lifetime. Many people will request a second test or go to a different healthcare provider for another HIV test because they believe that *HIV couldn't happen to me*. Let us explain what exactly occurs after you have an HIV test done, whether it is by swabbing the inside of your cheek, doing a finger stick, or having a tube of blood drawn.

There are two tests that need to be done before a diagnosis of HIV is confirmed. The first test, a preliminary test, confirms the presence of HIV antibodies. Such rapid testing, either by swabbing the inside of your cheek or by doing a finger stick, can give you a *preliminary result* in as little as five minutes. If positive, a blood sample will be sent to another lab to have a test, *Western blot*, performed. This second test will confirm the diagnosis of HIV. If your initial HIV screening test consisted of having a blood sample drawn, a preliminary test is run in the lab. If the preliminary test is positive, a second blood sample will be sent for a Western blot to confirm the diagnosis of HIV. These tests only confirm that you have HIV. They do not provide you or your healthcare provider with the information to determine your stage of disease.

It will usually take 1 to 2 weeks to get the test results.

Why Do People Get Tested for HIV?

There are many reasons for people to get tested for HIV. The Centers for Disease Control and Prevention recommend that anyone between the ages of 13 and 64 years be tested for HIV at least once as part of their routine healthcare. If they have *risk factors* that put them at risk for HIV, they should be tested for HIV annually.

Risk factors for HIV include the following:

- Unprotected sex with more than one partner
- Men having unprotected sex with other men
- Women having unprotected sex with men who have sex with other men
- Sharing drug paraphernalia (especially needles for intravenous drug use)
- Alcohol or drug use, making you more willing to engage in activities such as unprotected sex and put you at risk for acquiring HIV or other sexually transmitted infections
- Pregnancy (Pregnant women should be screened for HIV during 1st trimester and in the 3rd trimester if they have risk factors for acquiring HIV)

What Exactly Is the Difference between HIV and AIDS?

HIV, *human immunodeficiency virus*, is a virus that attacks your body's immune system. Viruses are very small particles that need host cells, such as plant, animal, or human cells, for their survival and replication. Some viruses that cause cold or flu enter your body and attack the respiratory or digestive cells. Your immune system, which helps fight infections, has learned to recognize these viruses, and when these viruses enter your body, the immune system begins producing antibodies to fight them.

HIV is passed from person to person when one comes in contact with body fluids through activities such as having unprotected sex (not using a condom) with someone who is HIV positive or sharing needles infected with HIV. When HIV enters a person's body, it attacks the cells of the immune system. HIV then uses these cells, called CD4 cells or T cells, to make new copies of itself. The new viruses infect other CD4 cells and thus multiply. HIV can make as many as 10 billion copies of itself each day. To fight off HIV, your body makes new CD4 cells daily. As the number of HIV in your body increases, more and more CD4 cells die trying to fight the viruses. The immune system becomes weaker and less able to fight other infections. Some people may experience flu-like symptoms such as fever, fatigue, or rash when they are first exposed to HIV, but many people have no symptoms at all.

Viruses like HIV can lie dormant, or sleep, for several years and not cause any symptoms. For that reason, people do not realize that they have been infected and may unknowingly pass on the infection to others. If untreated, HIV infection can lead to AIDS (*acquired immunodeficiency syndrome*). AIDS is advanced HIV disease and is characterized by a damaged immune system with a very low CD4 count, fewer than 200 cells, and related *opportunistic infections* and cancers. When you have these conditions, most life-threatening events occur. A list of AIDS-defining opportunistic infections and conditions are at the end of this chapter. HIV-related infections, including some opportunistic infections, are discussed in more detail later in this book.

The diagram on page 5 shows the life cycle of HIV. In the absence of any treatment, HIV makes millions of copies of itself daily and the virus destroys the immune system over time.

How HIV Is Transmitted

HIV can be transmitted in the following ways:

1. Having unprotected sex. This includes having anal, vaginal, or oral sex.
2. Sharing needles or syringes when doing drugs. There is also a risk of transmitting HIV from sharing pipes or other paraphernalia when there is a risk of blood being involved.
3. Receiving HIV-infected blood or blood products. The risk of acquiring HIV from blood or blood products is no longer a threat in the United States. Blood and blood products are routinely tested for HIV before being released for use. There may be a slight risk associated with receiving an organ donation.

A Service of the U.S. Department
of Health and Human Services

The HIV Life Cycle

1 **Binding and Fusion:** HIV begins its life cycle when it binds to a **CD4 receptor** and one of two **co-receptors** on the surface of a CD4⁺ **T-lymphocyte**. The virus then fuses with the host cell. After fusion, the virus releases RNA, its genetic material, into the host cell.

2 **Reverse Transcription:** An HIV enzyme called reverse transcriptase converts the single-stranded HIV RNA to double-stranded HIV DNA.

3 **Integration:** The newly formed HIV DNA enters the host cell's nucleus, where an HIV enzyme called integrase "hides" the HIV DNA within the host cell's own DNA. The integrated HIV DNA is called provirus. The provirus may remain inactive for several years, producing few or no new copies of HIV.

4 **Transcription:** When the host cell receives a signal to become active, the provirus uses a host enzyme called RNA polymerase to create copies of the HIV genomic material, as well as shorter strands of RNA called messenger RNA (mRNA). The mRNA is used as a blueprint to make long chains of HIV proteins.

5 **Assembly:** An HIV enzyme called protease cuts the long chains of HIV proteins into smaller individual proteins. As the smaller HIV proteins come together with copies of HIV's RNA genetic material, a new virus particle is assembled.

6 **Budding:** The newly assembled virus pushes out ("buds") from the host cell. During budding, the new virus steals part of the cell's outer envelope. This envelope, which acts as a covering, is studded with protein/sugar combinations called HIV glycoproteins. These HIV glycoproteins are necessary for the virus to bind CD4 and co-receptors. The new copies of HIV can now move on to infect other cells.

Terms Used in This Fact Sheet:

CD4 receptor: A protein present on the outside of infection-fighting white blood cells. CD4 receptors allow HIV to bind to and enter cells.

Co-receptor: In addition to binding a CD4 receptor, HIV must also bind either a CCR5 or CXCR4 co-receptor protein to get into a cell.

T-lymphocyte: A type of white blood cell that detects and fights foreign invaders of the body.

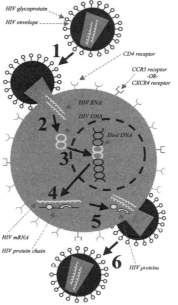

For more information:
Contact your doctor or an *AIDSinfo* Health Information Specialist at 1-800-448-0440 or **http://aidsinfo.nih.gov**.

May 2005

4. During pregnancy or childbirth, an HIV-infected woman could pass on HIV to her unborn child. If the HIV-positive woman is being treated for HIV, the risk of transmitting HIV to her infant is less than 2%. If the HIV-positive woman is not being treated for HIV, she has a 1 in 4 chance (or 25%) of passing on HIV to her infant.
5. HIV can also be transmitted to a baby in breast milk.

What Nurses Know...

You cannot get HIV through saliva, tears, sweat, urine, or feces. If there is blood in saliva, tears, sweat, urine, feces, or other bodily fluids, then it is the blood that may be a risk factor in transmission of HIV.

You can reduce the risk of transmitting or getting infected by HIV:

1. Know your HIV status by testing routinely
2. Know your sexual partner's HIV status
3. Use condoms if one or both of you are having sex with more than one person
4. Do not share needles
5. HIV-infected mothers should not breast-feed
6. If you are HIV positive:
   a) Tell every sexual partner or drug-using "buddy" that you have HIV
   b) Do not share needles
   c) Use latex condoms every time you have vaginal, anal, or oral sex
   d) Use birth control measures, as well as condoms, to avoid an accidental pregnancy
   e) Do not donate blood, semen, bone marrow, or other organs. Laws regarding organ donation are changing to allow people with HIV to receive an organ from someone who is also HIV infected. Talk to a representative of the organ donation bank in your area if you are interested in donating organs

What Nurses Know...

● ●

Always remember you cannot tell who is infected with HIV by looking at a person. Many people will look completely healthy. Many people do not realize they are infected. It takes an average of 8 to 15 years for symptoms of AIDS to develop after a person is infected with HIV.

AIDS-Defining Conditions

Below is a list of conditions, or infections, that constitute a diagnosis of AIDS, regardless of the CD4 cell count. Once a person has been diagnosed with AIDS, the diagnosis remains.

Bacterial infections

- *Mycobacterium avium* complex (also sometimes called *Mycobacterium avium-intracellulare*)
- Salmonella septicemia
- Tuberculosis
- Bacterial infections, multiple or recurrent

Viral infections

- Cytomegalovirus
- Herpes simplex; chronic ulcers or herpes bronchitis, pneumonitis, or esophagitis
- Progressive multifocal encephalopathy

Fungal infections

- Candidiasis of bronchi, trachea, or lungs
- Candidiasis of esophagus

- Coccidioidomycosis
- Cryptococcosis (cryptococcal meningitis)
- Histoplasmosis
- *Pneumocystis jiroveci* pneumonia

Protozoal infections

- Cryptosporidiosis
- Isosporiasis
- Toxoplasmosis

Malignancies

- Cervical cancer, invasive
- Kaposi's sarcoma
- Lymphomas

Other AIDS-defining conditions

- Pneumonia, recurrent
- Encephalopathy
- Wasting syndrome attributed to HIV

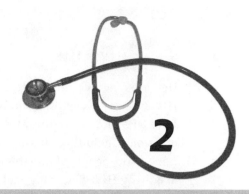

2

Now That I Know I Have HIV...What Happens Next?

Stages of Grieving, Denial, Depression, and Healthcare

The prenatal clinic made an appointment for me to see an HIV healthcare provider. I was really scared. I didn't think I could take any more bad news. I missed a lot of work because I couldn't stop crying and I didn't want my mom or anyone else to know what was going on. My husband and I just sort of went around like zombies. I missed two appointments before I finally went to see the HIV healthcare provider. Thank God I went. I saw a nurse practitioner who specializes in taking care of people who have HIV disease. She gave me a physical exam, she did a lot of laboratory tests, she asked me lots of questions, but most importantly, she answered all of mine. She let me cry, she held my hand. And she told me that there were medications. I could have a healthy baby–I could prevent giving HIV to my baby by taking medication. ALICIA, AGE 27

Denial is very common after you have been told that you have HIV. It is also very common for people who have been told they have HIV, or any life-threatening condition, to experience many emotions including denial, anger, fear, depression, and sadness. Many people blame themselves or their sexual partners for acquiring HIV. They may feel numb, confused, or overwhelmed. They may feel like their life is out of control or that they cannot make plans for the future. Some people may not be able to sleep or eat after being told they have HIV. They may even experience physical symptoms like feeling their heart race. These are all normal, and you need to allow yourself time to adjust to the diagnosis. You may need to delay making important decisions until you have acquired knowledge about the disease and a plan for improving or maintaining your health. You may need to talk to your provider about seeking treatment for some of your physical symptoms, like insomnia or anxiety, or discuss the need to follow up with a mental health counselor. Remember, being told you have HIV does not mean you have AIDS. It is no longer the death sentence it was 30 years ago. Today, there are many medications available to treat HIV and AIDS.

Who knows that you have HIV. Obviously, the physician, nurse, or testing counselor who performed the test or gave you the results knows that you have HIV. But there are also other people who know your test results that you may not have thought about or even know that they are given the results, such as the lab personnel who ran the test or staff at your insurance company. HIV is also a *reportable condition*, which means it is one of the several diseases that are considered to be of public health importance. There are laws that mandate healthcare providers and laboratories to report these types of diseases to the local or state health department. Many of these diseases, such as HIV, also must be reported to the Centers for Disease Control and Prevention. HIV is considered a sexually transmitted infection (STI). In the case of STIs, in many states, there are workers who will attempt to notify the people who might have been exposed to HIV or other STIs through sexual contact or by sharing needles.

The state workers will not identify you as the source but will tell your contacts that they may have been exposed to an STI. This reporting is necessary so that your contacts will be tested early for HIV and can receive appropriate care if they are HIV infected or have another STI.

We have discussed who might know that you have HIV. Now let us discuss the laws that protect you. There are laws that prevent healthcare workers from telling anyone, other than the mandated health departments, about your HIV status without your consent. There are laws that prevent organizations, such as employers and housing agencies, from discriminating against people with HIV. You do not have to tell your employer you have HIV.

For more information about your legal rights, you can contact your local legal aid office or find information at HIV Law and Policy at www.hivlawandpolicy.org.

Now That You Know You Have HIV, Here Are Some Important First Steps

1. Educate yourself about HIV and AIDS. The more you know about HIV, the better decisions you can make now and in the future. Your local health department or public library may have resources available. Be careful when viewing HIV information over the Internet. They can provide misleading information. There is a list of reputable Web sites in the Resources section at the end of the book.

2. Find a healthcare provider who has training/expertise in the management and treatment of HIV/AIDS. If you have a family or primary care provider (PCP), ask him/her for a recommendation. You may also want to contact your local health department or AIDS Service Organization and ask for a list of experienced HIV healthcare providers in your area. Your insurance company may also direct you to an infectious disease specialist. If you do not have health insurance, your local

health department will also be able to tell you if there are federally funded programs available in your area. These Ryan White programs may provide primary care, case management, mental health or substance-abuse counseling, antiretrovirals (HIV medications), housing, or other services. HIV care and Ryan White programs will be discussed later in this chapter.

3. Coping with the diagnosis. If you feel that you are unable to cope with the stress, if you are using drugs or alcohol to cope, or if coping strategies you have used in the past are not working, you may need to seek help from a mental health therapist or counselor. Again, you can ask your PCP or local health department for a referral or assistance in finding counselors in your area. Mental health counseling may also be provided through Ryan White services in your area.

4. Who to tell. Adding to your stress in coping with a diagnosis of HIV may be your uncertainty in sharing this with friends or family. Most of us turn to family members and friends in times of stress for help with making decisions and for comfort. Think about whom you want to tell—and why you want this person(s) to know about your diagnosis. They may express fears or concerns about HIV. Keep in mind that their fears and concerns are due to their lack of knowledge. If you have begun educating yourself about HIV, you will be better prepared to answer their questions. Friends and family members may also need time to think about and process the news of your HIV diagnosis. While this may be difficult for you, remember your own feelings while being given the diagnosis and allow them this time. Remember, you are still the same person you were before you were told you had HIV.

People you must or should tell include people with whom you have had sex or have shared needles. It is important that they know so that they can be tested for HIV.

You also need to tell your healthcare providers. This might include your PCP if he or she is unaware, dentists, ophthalmologists or optometrists (eye doctors), or other healthcare workers.

All healthcare workers should use gloves and other protective garb to decrease the risk of exposure, but they should be aware of your HIV diagnosis to ensure they follow appropriate procedures. Importantly for you, healthcare providers should also have this information to thoroughly and accurately provide care to you.

Taking the Next Step: Seeing an Experienced HIV Healthcare Provider

Making an appointment to see an HIV healthcare provider often makes the HIV diagnosis *real*. Many people facing this step will postpone that appointment as long as possible. Their reasons are that they feel fine, they do not have any symptoms, they do not want to miss work, or they do not want their family to know ... the list can go on and on. This is part of the denial process after someone is told they have HIV. For some people denial can last months or even years. A few people may wait until they do have symptoms and then the panic of having HIV starts all over again.

Take a deep breath, make that appointment, and keep it! Only by taking this step you will get the answers you need. Then you and the provider can begin creating a healthcare plan that is right for you to fight HIV and maintain or improve your health.

The first appointment with an HIV specialist will include many of the procedures you might have experienced with other healthcare appointments. A nurse or technician will take your *vital signs* (temperature, pulse, respirations, blood pressure) and measurements, such as height and weight. You will be asked if you have any allergies to medications or foods and if you are currently taking any medications. Later, the HIV specialist will want to discuss your health history, including other health conditions you might have, infectious agents you might have been exposed to, immunization/vaccination history, mental health history, and your family history.

Your healthcare provider will want to know if you have been tested for HIV in the past and if you can remember having flu-like symptoms between your last negative test and your positive test. Flu-like

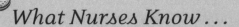

What Nurses Know...

It is very common to forget information when you go to healthcare visits. To help prepare you for this visit, before your appointment, write down all the medications you are currently taking, as much of your health history as you know (previous or current health conditions, surgeries, and immunization history), and your family health history, such as a history of heart disease on your father's side.

symptoms may be caused by recently being exposed to HIV. If you just recently had or currently have flu symptoms, your provider may consider starting you on antiretroviral therapy immediately.

Because HIV is transmitted through unprotected sex or by sharing needles, your HIV specialist will also want to discuss your risk factors for acquiring HIV. This will include a discussion of your substance abuse and sexual history. This is not meant to embarrass you, but to make certain that you are not putting yourself or other people at risk of acquiring other STIs or HIV. Part of your treatment plan will be how to decrease behaviors that put you or others at risk and how to increase behaviors that protect you, such as always using condoms when having sex or not sharing needles.

This provider will also want to review your *past medical* and *medication history* by asking you questions about

- Other chronic health conditions you might have (such as diabetes or high blood pressure)
- Sexually transmitted infections or diseases (STIs or STDs) you have had in the past (such as gonorrhea, syphilis, herpes, chlamydia)
- Infectious diseases such as tuberculosis or tuberculosis exposure
- Hepatitis and if you have received immunizations against hepatitis A and B

- Previous surgeries or hospitalizations
- Mental health and mental health treatment
- Substance abuse and substance-abuse treatment
- Smoking history
- Women's health history such as
  - Date of last pap smear, past history of abnormal pap smears
  - Last menstrual period and discussion about the usual number of days between periods and how heavy the flow
  - Pregnancy history
- All prior vaccinations, including tetanus
- All current medications, including over-the-counter medications and herbal and nutritional supplements
- Previous primary care history. If possible, take a written list to this appointment with the names and addresses of healthcare providers you have seen in the past. It may help for this new provider to have your old medical records to have a full understanding of your history
- Previous screenings
- If you have been treated for HIV in the past
  - Previous antiretroviral history
  - Medications to prevent or treat *opportunistic infections*

Your HIV healthcare provider will also want to discuss your social history, including employment, housing, support system, family, pets, travel history, and history of violence. It is important for your provider to understand your responsibilities and any issues that might impact your care or your ability to successfully take medications to fight HIV. Your HIV provider will also want to assess your knowledge about HIV.

Your provider will want to review any symptoms you might be experiencing and will ask about your overall health and then about specific areas. The discussion may be in any order but will target the following areas

- Overall: fevers, chills, night sweats, fatigue, loss of appetite, or weight loss

- Head/ears/eyes/neck/throat: any changes in vision or hearing, headaches, sinus discomfort, sores or lesions in your mouth (including your tongue), sore throat, or difficulty or pain when swallowing
- Lymph nodes: history or current problems with swollen or painful lymph nodes
- Lungs: shortness of breath, at rest or with activity; cough; sputum; or phlegm
- Heart: chest pain, feeling like your heart is racing
- Stomach: nausea, vomiting, diarrhea, constipation, pain
- Genitals and urinary: burning, frequency, discomfort or urgency when urinating; sores, warts, lesions on penis or vagina; tenderness, bleeding, or discharge from penis or vagina; and bleeding from rectum
- Skin: sores, rashes, abnormal bruising, or lumps
- Mental health: depression, anxiety, insomnia, forgetfulness, and changes in mood

Your HIV healthcare provider will also perform a thorough "head to toe" *physical exam* focusing on

- Ears, eyes, nose, mouth, and throat
- Lymph nodes
- Heart: listening and noting the rate and rhythm, or any other abnormal sounds
- Lungs: listening to your lungs as you breathe in and out
- Abdomen: feeling for masses or organ enlargement, measuring your liver
- Neurology: testing the reflexes and sensations in your legs and feet
- Skin: looking at your skin and noting any sores, rashes, abnormal bruising, or lumps
- Feet and legs: checking to see if you have any swelling
- Women: may also have a pelvic exam and pap smear, rectal exam, and breast exam done at this time or you may ask your provider to wait to do at another appointment
- Men: penis, testicular, rectal, and prostate exams

At the end of your "head to toe" exam, your HIV healthcare provider will want to discuss the initial physicial exam and assessment and plan for your ongoing care. Your provider will want to discuss some or all of the following:

- How HIV works in your body and how your HIV provider can determine how much damage has been done to the immune system and currently how active the virus is
- How HIV is transmitted and the ways you can decrease risk to yourself and your partners
- The importance of maintaining your health: good nutrition, exercise, sleep, and all the things you hear that you should be doing. They really are important!
- Smoking (either stopping or decreasing)
- Practice good hand-washing
- The importance of keeping appointments
- Symptoms that should be reported
- Plan for having children, if applicable
- The availability of community services, such as Ryan White case management, support groups, and other community programs
- The lab tests that your provider would like to order at this first visit. It is important to have these done soon so that at your next visit your HIV healthcare provider can discuss the stage of HIV, if you need to consider starting antiretrovirals, and if there are other health conditions that need to be addressed
- Your next follow-up visit should be scheduled prior to leaving this appointment. You should also receive information (ask for it, if necessary) about how to contact your provider between office visits if you have symptoms or questions

Lab assessment and diagnostic testing:

- HIV antibody testing may be repeated, unless documentation of a previous positive HIV test result
- Complete blood count
- CD4+ T cell count (immune panel)

- HIV viral load (analysis of plasma ribonucleic acid levels by polymerase chain reaction)
- HIV resistance testing (genotype tests should be done for new HIV diagnosis or if you have not started antiretrovirals)
- Comprehensive metabolic panel (this includes liver tests and kidney tests)
- Hepatitis tests (for hepatitis A, B, and C)
- Lipid (cholesterol) test: if you are not fasting, this should be done at a later date, preferably before your next appointment
- Screening for STIs: gonorrhea, chlamydia, and syphilis; the test for gonorrhea and chlamydia may be done by urine collection
- Urine screening
- Screening for tuberculosis
- Pregnancy testing, if applicable

Ryan White HIV/AIDS Programs

The Ryan White CARE (Comprehensive AIDS Resources Emergency) Act was first enacted in 1990 and has been reauthorized several times since then by the federal government. The purpose of the CARE Act is to provide health and social services to those living with HIV who do not have private or public health insurance, have inadequate health coverage, or lack the financial means to get the HIV healthcare they need. This federally funded program works with states, cities, and local community-based organizations to provide HIV-related services to more than 500,000 people annually. The majority of Ryan White funding goes to support HIV primary medical care and HIV support services, which could include medical case management, oral/dental care, mental health or substance-abuse treatment, AIDS Drug Assistance Program, and a variety of other services. The programs are broken down into parts: Parts A, B, C, D, and F. The following information about each part is taken from the HRSA Web site, www.hrsa.gov.

Part A provides emergency assistance to Eligible Metropolitan Areas and Transitional Grant Areas that are most severely affected by the HIV/AIDS epidemic.

Part B provides grants to all 50 States, the District of Columbia, Puerto Rico, Guam, the U.S. Virgin Islands, and five U.S. Pacific territories or associated jurisdictions.

Part C provides comprehensive primary healthcare in an outpatient setting for people living with HIV disease.

Part D provides family-centered care involving outpatient or ambulatory care for women, infants, children, and youth with HIV/AIDS.

Part F provides funds a variety of programs:

1. The Special Projects of National Significance Program grants funds for innovative models of care and supports the development of effective delivery systems for HIV care.
2. The AIDS Education and Training Centers Program supports a network of 11 regional centers and several national centers that conduct targeted, multidisciplinary education and training programs for healthcare providers treating people living with HIV/AIDS.
3. The Dental Programs provide additional funding for oral healthcare for people with HIV.
4. The Minority AIDS Initiative provides funding to evaluate and address the disproportionate impact of HIV/AIDS on African Americans and other minorities.

Working with a Ryan White Medical Case Manager

Ryan White Case Management is a federally funded voluntary program designed to improve the longevity and quality of life of persons living with HIV. Ryan White case managers can provide a variety of services to assist individuals and families infected, or affected, by HIV.

Ryan White case managers are able to help people with HIV access care and coordinate care among several healthcare providers. They will provide education and help persons living with HIV access antiretroviral medications for the treatment of HIV disease. You can contact your local public health department for information about Ryan White programs available in your area or go online to http://hab.hrsa.gov.

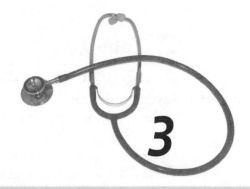

3

Managing HIV: The Basics

In the beginning, I couldn't remember what they told me in the clinic. I didn't understand what my labs meant or why I needed to be stuck so much for tests. Now I write everything down and my provider always makes sure I understand what is going on. SAM, AGE 42

Your first visit with an HIV expert was probably pretty overwhelming! You may not remember all the people you came into contact with that day or know what to expect the next time you keep a provider appointment. You actually have a whole team of health professionals to help you learn to live a healthy life with HIV. Let us review a little bit about the people you might have met during your first visit with an HIV provider and whom you might meet in the future.

As mentioned in Chapter 2, your HIV provider could be a medical doctor (MD), a doctor of osteopathy (DO), a nurse practitioner (NP), or a physician's assistant (PA). All these health professionals may specialize in treating persons with HIV. NPs are nurses who have obtained an advanced degree in nursing and work in collaboration with a physician or physicians. PAs are typically not nurses but have a bachelor's degree in another field and then obtain additional education to become a PA. PAs work with physicians. If you have other health conditions or your HIV is very advanced, an NP or PA may refer you to an MD or DO to assist in or manage your care.

Besides your healthcare provider, there are other health professionals who may be part of your healthcare team. Your team may include nurses, peer educators, social workers or case managers, pharmacists, dietitians or nutritionists, counselors, and receptionists.

Nurses: Registered nurses have 2 to 4 years of education and graduate from an approved school of nursing; licensed practical nurses and licensed vocational nurses have 1 year of education and graduate from an approved program. These nurses must also pass an exam to be able to practice in individual states. Nursing assistants or nursing technicians would usually have attended a hospital-based or certification program.

Registered nurses and licensed practical nurses who work in clinics or doctors' offices are an important part of your team. They can provide more detailed education about HIV or other health conditions, discuss your lab results, advise about creating a healthcare plan, and answer questions you may have following your provider's visit.

Nurses usually talk to patients when they call about health concerns or medication issues. It is important that you have all the information available to give them, so that they have an accurate understanding of your needs and can relay that information to the provider.

Peer educators (counselors or advocates): Peers are people who live with HIV and have received additional training to help provide education to others who are also HIV positive. They can provide basic HIV education and information about local community resources and help newly diagnosed patients navigate a complex medical system. Peers may be a part of the team at your provider's office or clinic, or they may be part of an AIDS Service Organization (ASO), such as case management or housing. Ask your provider or nurse if there are peers in the clinic, or contact your local health department and ask if there are peers in your area.

Social workers or case managers: Case managers or social workers can provide education about HIV and help with information about, or referrals to, housing, insurance, legal issues, mental health or substance-abuse counseling, and AIDS drug assistance programs. They may be located within your provider's clinic or at an ASO. If your provider does not have a social worker or case manager on-site, you can contact your local health department for information about these services.

Pharmacists: Whether your provider has a pharmacist working in the clinic or you have contact with a pharmacist at your local drug store, pharmacists are an important part of your healthcare team. They can provide information about the medications you take, inform you if there are drugs you are prescribed that may not work well together, or inform you if you should take medications at a certain time with or without food. It is preferable that you use only one pharmacy for filling your prescriptions so that the pharmacist has a complete picture of the medications you take. It is risky to your health if you see more than one provider and also use more than one pharmacy. For that reason, you should always carry a complete list of all the medications, including over-the-counter medications and any herbal or alternative therapies that you take, and share that information with your provider(s) and pharmacist(s). Many cities may also have HIV specialty pharmacies such as BioScrip. Even chain drug stores, such as Walgreens, may have pharmacies with HIV-experienced pharmacists and provide HIV specialty services. Discuss using a specialty drug store with your provider, nurse, or case manager.

Dietitians or nutritionists: Some providers or clinics may employ a dietitian or nutritionist to help clients maintain a healthy diet. Or, if you need that service, your provider may refer you to a dietitian at a local hospital. Nutrition is an important component for maintaining optimal health. Even if you do not need to see a dietitian or nutritionist at this time, look for information on maintaining a healthy diet.

Counselors, for mental health or substance abuse: At some time, you may need to seek help for depression, anxiety, or other mental health issues or help with reducing your dependency on alcohol or drugs, either recreational or prescription pain meds. Your provider or one of your healthcare team members may refer you to a counselor to help with these issues. Your counselor will become a part of your team to help you achieve your health goals.

Receptionist: Do not forget this important member of your healthcare team; the receptionist can help you set up your appointments and provide you with information for other referrals. The receptionist is also the first person you talk to if you need to contact your provider about issues regarding your health or medications.

What Nurses Know . . .

Your healthcare team also includes people in your life who you trust to help provide emotional support while you learn to live with HIV. These very important members include family, friends, or members of your faith community. They can help encourage you during the difficult times, encourage you to keep health-related appointments, and remind you to take medications.

Steps to Maintain Your Health

Before you were diagnosed with HIV, you might only have seen a healthcare provider when you were ill. That is all going to change now. It is important that you routinely see your provider two to four times a year. You will see your provider more frequently if you are starting or changing HIV medications, or if you are having symptoms related to HIV or your medications.

What Nurses Know...

Making and keeping your appointments are critical to creating a good relationship with your provider. You will want to have up-to-date information about your labs, discuss any symptoms you might have experienced since the last visit, and update or revise the plan you have created to maintain or improve your health. It is advisable to always take a calendar with you to your provider visits so that you can easily schedule and track your next appointment and when you should have blood drawn for testing.

As you know, HIV can lie dormant, or sleep, for several years and you may not have any symptoms. There is so much to do everyday, and it is very tempting to miss an appointment with your provider if you are feeling fine. Most of us grew up thinking we only need to see a provider when we are sick. How strange to go when we feel well. However, even if you do not have symptoms, HIV can still be damaging your immune system. Only by seeing your provider regularly and having lab tests done will you know your health status. If you are taking HIV medications, the lab tests also tell you and the provider if the medications are working the way they should.

Missing or frequently rescheduling appointments may indicate to the provider that you are not serious about your health and jeopardize your ability to get an appointment if/when you experience a serious health issue.

Having an honest and trusting relationship with your provider is vital to achieving your optimal health. You must be able to talk openly with your provider about all aspects of your health and lifestyle. Only then will the two of you have a partnership that works together to make good decisions.

The initial visit with a provider typically takes about an hour. Further visits are usually much shorter. Because you may only have 15 minutes or so with your provider, you need to make the most of that visit! Plan ahead. Keep a notebook and write down questions, concerns, or symptoms between visits. Before a visit with your provider, decide which member of your healthcare team can best answer your questions. You may want to discuss results of lab tests, new symptoms, or medication side effects with your provider. Your pharmacist or nurse may be able to discuss how or when to take your medications. Your nurse or peer educator might be able to explain what certain lab tests are and why they are done. Rank your questions and ensure that your three highest-ranking questions are answered before you leave your provider's office. If necessary, make an appointment with a nurse, peer educator, or case manager to further discuss your health concerns.

Your healthcare provider will also want to know *all* medications you are taking, including any over-the-counter or herbal medications. This is especially important if you are seeing more

What Nurses Know . . .

At the end of each visit to the healthcare provider, you should always repeat to the provider the key points of your discussion to ensure that you both have the same understanding of what was said during your visit. It is important that you clearly understand any new health information and changes to your health plan. This is also an opportunity for the provider to answer any follow-up questions or provide clearer information.

than one provider, including a mental health provider. Ensure that your provider has an updated list of your medications at every visit. You may want to carry a card that lists all your current medications and allergies.

Because many members of your healthcare team will be providing you with education and information, it is important that you all agree on the healthcare/treatment plan that *you* are most comfortable with. Your provider and your team members can provide you with the information and recommend what they feel is in your best interest, but in the end, it is *your* decision to take the medication or follow their recommendations.

Make your health a priority and seek out the answers to your questions. You have a team to help you, but only you can lead the team to achieve *your* goals.

Have your labs tests done on a routine basis: CD4 counts and HIV viral loads are important markers that monitor the status of your immune system and if the antiretroviral (ARV) medications you are taking are "working" as they should. These labs, as well as other important labs, are discussed later in this chapter. Laboratory testing (blood and/or urine) is typically done every 1 to 6 months depending on where you are in your disease progression and how long you have been taking a stable regimen of ARV medications. For individuals who are early in their course of HIV treatment or have been switched to a new regimen of ARV medications, lab work will be done more often. Once you are on a stable regimen of ARV treatment, lab tests are typically done less often. For most people living with HIV, on average, lab tests are done about every 3 to 4 months.

Take your medicine correctly, even if you are feeling well. Remember that HIV is killing healthy CD4 cells even when you do not feel sick. You should take your prescribed medicine for any health condition correctly so that you and your provider can more easily determine the cause of abnormal lab values or health-related concerns, such as blood pressure that is higher than normal. Remember to always be honest with your provider about what medicines you are and/or are not taking. Telling the provider what you think they want to hear does not help you, and really does not make them happy. Working together, honestly, is very important to maintain or improve your health.

Get immunizations or vaccinations (shots) to prevent other infections, such as pneumonia or hepatitis A or B. At your first visit, you should have had lab work done to determine if you have been exposed to hepatitis A or B. If you do not have immunity to hepatitis A or B, you should also be vaccinated for that virus. You should also be vaccinated for flu yearly and be sure to keep current on your tetanus vaccination.

If you plan to travel to other countries, you will need to find out if additional vaccinations are required. You can contact your county health department for assistance in finding information about vaccination requirements and where you can obtain them. You can also check out two sites on the CDC.gov page about vaccinations: http://www.cdc.gov/vaccines/ or http://wwwnc.cdc.gov/travel/page/vaccinations.htm.

See a dentist every 6 months to have your teeth and gums examined and cleaned. Brush your teeth at least twice a day. Good oral hygiene is important. Mouth infections are common in people living with HIV. Examine your mouth daily for white patches or bumps on your tongue, gums, or roof of your mouth.

What Nurses Know...

Wash your Hands! *Hand washing is one of the most important ways to prevent an infection from occurring. Wash your hands before and after you eat, after using the toilet, and after being around someone who has a cold or flu. Encourage people around you to wash their hands often to avoid passing on their germs. Remember that someone else has probably handled everything you touch.*

Get healthy habits: Eat healthy, nutritious food. This will help keep you strong, give you energy, and keep your weight within a normal range. Many foods also boost your immunity and help the body protect itself. This information will be discussed in more detail in Chapter 4. Exercise regularly, but moderately, to maintain muscle. Remember to get enough sleep and rest. This can sometimes be much harder to do than it sounds. Your body and mind need rest to function well and to focus on daily matters, but anxiety, fear, depression, pain, and other aspects of life make it very difficult to take enough rest. See Chapter 4 for more discussion on this topic and some tips for getting the sleep you need.

If you smoke, drink, or do drugs…QUIT! Again, easier to say than to do, but there are good reasons to limit their toxic effects on your body. Smokers have more secretions in their lungs than nonsmokers. These secretions make it easier for microorganisms to grow in your lungs and cause pneumonia and infection. Alcohol and drugs, such as cocaine, marijuana, and amphetamines, are dangerous for persons living with HIV. They can lower your resistance to infections, interfere with your medicines, and cause problems with your nutrition. We will discuss these in more detail in Chapter 4, but you should seriously consider talking to a member of your healthcare team about counseling or other options.

Attitude is everything: There has been much research done about the effects of attitude in managing a chronic health condition. If you feel depressed or overwhelmed, talk to a member of your healthcare team about mental health counseling or support groups in your area. Remember, you are the same person that you were before you knew that you had HIV, with the same hopes, dreams, and aspirations. Keep moving forward.

Keep track of your health information: You probably left your first provider visit feeling pretty overwhelmed and struggling to remember everything you were told, which is very common. For that reason it is important for you to find a method to keep track of your health information. You might have noticed during your first visit that you had difficulty giving information about your childhood immunizations, or could not remember the name of a medicine you took a few years ago that caused a rash. It did not seem important at the time, but now you have discovered that it might be important in the future.

Some people keep their health information in a folder or a box. Others may organize it in a notebook. Whatever works for you is all that matters, but here is a breakdown of what information you need to keep of your health history (as far back as you can remember or have records). Update this history after each visit with your provider:

1. Allergies to both medications and food, including the symptoms you experience when taking or eating them
2. Health conditions and dates they were diagnosed, including date of HIV diagnosis
3. Surgeries
4. Medications, including dates started and stopped. This is especially important when keeping track of your HIV medication history. You will want to record any side effects experienced and why a medication was stopped, and whether it was stopped by you or your provider
5. Vaccinations and immunizations. It is easy to forget about when your last tetanus shot was or to get a yearly flu shot. For that reason, keeping track of vaccinations and immunizations is very important
6. Lab results. Important information to track related to HIV would be CD4 counts, HIV viral loads, and HIV resistance tests. If you also have other conditions, such as diabetes, you will want to keep track of fasting blood sugars and hemoglobin A1C. You may also want to keep track of abnormal lab results, such as for liver or kidney, even if there is no clear diagnosis related to them. If you change providers or are hospitalized, they may want or need that information.

Even though you have HIV, you have to work to keep your whole body healthy. There are screenings that should be done annually and others you will need to do as you get older. A schedule of general health screenings for both men and women are provided at the end of this chapter.

Some of the steps we have listed will be easy to incorporate into your life, but some steps will require more effort or willpower to be incorporated. Any healthy change, no matter how small, will make a difference. It may take time to see progress, but patience and perseverance will lead to rewards. Incorporating these healthy steps into your life will not only help manage a chronic health condition but also help improve your overall health. Some of the steps are discussed in detail later in this book.

Signs and symptoms to be reported to your provider: Earlier in this chapter we discussed the importance of keeping regular appointments with your provider, even when you are feeling well. Now we need to discuss the times between your provider appointments when you do not feel well or experience symptoms that are out of the ordinary. It is confusing and sometimes frightening when you do not know if you are experiencing something serious or just a common cold. This is especially true if your immune system is badly damaged. You should also track these symptoms. You may notice a pattern when some of these symptoms occur, which could help you and your provider in determining the cause and the treatment. Here is a list of symptoms that should be reported to your provider:

- Diarrhea. Having more than five watery or loose stools per day. Until the cause of the diarrhea is determined, try to avoid dairy products, spices, fresh fruits, and food high in fat. Also avoid alcohol and products that have caffeine, such as coffee, tea, and soda pop
- Weight loss or loss of appetite. If you have a scale, write down your weight once a week or after each visit with your provider. Be sure to bring your weight diary with you. Try to eat smaller, more frequent meals, five to six times a day
- Trouble or pain when swallowing
- White patches or sores in or around your mouth

- Fever—lasting more than 2 days. If you have a thermometer, check your temperature two to three times per day and write it down along with the time that you checked your temperature. Ensure to take your fever diary to your provider appointment. Also, drink plenty of fluids, especially water, and get lots of rest
- A new cough—even if you are not coughing up phlegm. If you are coughing up phlegm, be sure to tell your provider the color of it. Let the provider know if you also have a fever
- Shortness of breath. When you visit the provider, ensure you tell him/her if the shortness of breath occurs while you are resting, moving about, or both. If you experience shortness of breath doing your usual daily activities, try to increase your rest periods. Plan activities so that you can take fewer steps
- Headaches or dizziness
- Changes in vision, including blurred vision or seeing "floaters"
- Trouble remembering things

It can be confusing to know if the above symptoms are really serious enough to be reported to the provider. If you typically have allergy symptoms in the spring, you may be used to having a cough or "sinus" headaches. You may usually have diarrhea after eating salad. However, if the symptoms seem different or last longer than usual, you should report them to your provider. Only you know about your body and what is normal for you.

It is always better to contact your provider during normal business hours. Waiting until your provider is unavailable may cause you to make unnecessary visits to an emergency department. Emergency departments are often the busiest places in a hospital, so we encourage you to seek medical care during office hours, when possible.

During your first or second visit with your provider, you should discuss what to do if you become ill after clinic hours or on the weekend. Your provider may have an answering service or refer to another provider who routinely covers weekends. You should ask what hospital your provider prefers you to use if you need urgent medical care.

What Nurses Know ...

Having a plan in place for emergencies will make you feel more comfortable about what to do in the future. Ensure that you keep that information in a handy area and that at least one other person knows where to find it if they need to contact someone for you. Also, keep a list readily available of your current medications and any allergies that you have. This will make it easier for you to answer questions correctly if you are talking to someone other than your usual provider.

If you are experiencing some of the symptoms we just discussed, here are some tips that may help:

Loss of appetite

- Eat smaller, more frequent meals
- Drink protein shakes or smoothies between meals

Nausea/vomiting

- Avoid greasy or spicy foods
- Avoid foods with a strong odor
- Eat bland or mild foods
- Avoid foods that are hot or cold; eat foods that are at moderate temperature
- Eat several small meals per day, rather than three large meals
- Avoid drinking fluids with meals
- If you have had more than one episode of nausea and vomiting in the past 30 days, keep a diary of your weight
- Talk to your provider if vomiting lasts more than 2 days, or if you become dizzy or weak

Diarrhea

- Drink plenty of decaffeinated fluids
- Avoid greasy, fried, and spicy foods
- Avoid high-fiber foods
- Limit dairy products, such as milk and ice cream
- Eat bland foods, such as rice, bananas, and bread

Mouth sores

- Avoid spicy and salty foods
- Avoid citrus fruits, such as oranges and grapefruits
- Avoid hard foods, such as chips or popcorn
- Eat soft, moist, smooth foods
- Eat foods that are cold or at room temperature
- Use a straw to drink liquids

Fatigue

- Keep your kitchen stocked with foods that are easy to prepare
- Eat frozen or canned foods
- Fix simple meals or snacks
- Ask friends or family to cook for you
- Use paper cups and plates, if necessary
- Talk to your provider or case manager about agencies that bring meals to the door

Understanding Your Lab Tests

Lab tests are another type of examination—usually of your blood, urine, or other body fluids, such as sputum—that are done in a laboratory to help provide a better understanding of your overall health. These tests are done to monitor the effects of HIV infection and if medications you are taking are working as well as anticipated. Certain tests can also indicate if there are complications from the HIV infection, the medications you are taking, or other health conditions. Along with signs and symptoms you may report to your provider, they help create a better understanding of your health status. For this reason, it is important that you understand some of the basic, routine lab tests that your provider will want to have performed. You should also include results from these tests in your *health information record.*

CD4 cells or T-cells are a type of white blood cell that makes up the bulk of the body's immune defense system. They are the body's first defense against invaders, such as viruses, including HIV. Unfortunately, CD4 cells are also what HIV prefers to attack and infect. HIV is able to use the CD4's DNA to replicate, or make more copies of itself.

CD4 counts are done at your first visit (baseline), 2 to 8 weeks after you start HIV medications, routinely every 3 to 4 months if you are taking HIV medications, or every 6 months if you are not taking HIV medications. CD4 counts will typically increase if the HIV medications are effective, with the goal of the medication being to increase CD4 count as much as possible. If your CD4 count is under 200, the goal would be for it to increase the CD4 count to 200. Most opportunistic infections (OIs) occur when the CD4 count is less than 200.

A normal CD4 count varies between 500 to 1,500 cells per cubic millimeter of blood. Everyone's CD4 cell count varies a little, which is normal. However, CD4 count will decline below 500, over time, if HIV is not treated or if the HIV medications are no longer working. As your CD4 count gets lower (especially below 200 cells), the greater the chances of getting infections. A decline in CD4 cell count may indicate that HIV infection is progressing and the immune system is getting weaker. However, if your CD4 count has been within the normal range, one low CD4 count alone does not mean that HIV has seriously damaged your immune system or you have progressed to AIDS. If you have been ill with a cold or other illness, your immune system could be weakened from fighting that infection. A second CD4 count taken before your next provider visit will give more information, such as if this is a trend and if additional steps need to be taken. If your CD4 count continues to decline, you and your provider will need to discuss starting or changing your ARV medications or adding medications to prevent OIs. OIs typically occur when the immune system is not working well and the CD4 count is below 200 cells.

HIV viral load is the amount of HIV in the blood. Remember how we discussed that HIV makes copies of itself? That replication is also used to describe the amount of virus in the blood. Depending on the HIV activity, the viral load may be high, over 100,000 copies, or low, less than 10,000 copies. People with high viral loads are more likely to also have a decrease in CD4 cell count. Consequently, HIV may progress faster when the viral load is high than when it is low. When you are taking HIV medications, the goal of treatment is to decrease the number of HIV copies to less than 50, sometimes called *undetectable.* Having an undetectable viral load does not mean that you no longer have HIV, but HIV medications are working as they should and the viral load has been effectively suppressed.

- HIV viral loads are typically done at the same time when CD4 cell counts are scheduled: the first visit (baseline), 2 to 8 weeks after you start HIV medications, routinely every 3 to 4 months if you are taking HIV medications, or every 6 months if you are not taking HIV medications
- The viral load measurements together with the CD4 count are used by the HIV healthcare provider to determine when someone with HIV should initiate treatment for HIV disease with ARVs. After you have started taking ARVs, the viral load measurement indicates the effectiveness of the medications and whether or not they are "working" as they should. What you want is for the viral load to decrease, and for the CD4 cell count to increase. Usually, the viral load will decrease within weeks of starting ARV or when changing ARV medications. The goal is to decrease the viral load to what is called "undetectable" levels (<50 or <20 copies, depending on the laboratory used)

- The CD4 cell count and HIV viral load (also called HIV polymerase chain reaction test) are two very important lab tests that help determine how healthy your immune system is. Your provider will use both these lab measurements to help determine when you need to start ARV medications and, if you are taking ARV medications, how well they are working. These test results are also important for you to track your *health information record.* Ask your provider or nurse for copies of your test result or write them down before you leave the office or clinic

HIV resistance tests are done when the CD4 count and HIV viral load indicate that the HIV medications are no longer working. There are many reasons why HIV medications fail to work as they should, and these are discussed in another chapter. When the HIV viral load starts to increase, your provider will be concerned that the medications are no longer working and may order a test to determine if the virus has become resistant to the medications. The HIV may have mutated or changed its genetic structure, which allows it to make copies of itself, despite the HIV medications.

There are two types of resistance tests that can be done: genotype testing and phenotype testing. Both are blood tests that can help determine which HIV medications the virus will not respond to. You should write down the dates of any HIV resistance tests you have done in your health information record.

- Genotype testing looks for HIV mutations in a blood sample and then compares them to a list of mutations known to cause resistance to specific HIV medications
- Phenotype testing takes a sample of blood and divides it into many tubes. Each tube is then exposed to a different HIV medication. This testing can tell you exactly which drug your virus will be resistant to. This test is more costly and takes a longer period of time to receive results

More information about HIV drug resistance can be found in Chapter 5.

Complete blood count provides measurement of red blood cells, white blood cells, and platelets. Abnormally high or low results could indicate infection, certain diseases, or toxicities caused by drugs or treatments.

Liver function tests are done to detect liver damage or liver disease. If you are taking certain HIV medications or medications for other diseases, liver function tests may be done once or twice a year.

Kidney function tests are done to evaluate how well the kidneys are working. Diabetes and high blood pressure can damage your kidneys, as well as some medications.

Each time you discuss your lab measurements with your healthcare provider, be certain to ask if there are any abnormal results you should know about. While your provider may not know the cause, it is important that you record them in your *health information record* and include them in your conversation with your provider in the future.

On the next pages, we have included examples of health records and general screening guidelines for men and women. There are also chapters in the book devoted entirely to men's and women's health.

Medication Record

A medication record should be used to keep track of all medications you are taking. Remember to include any over-the-counter medications and herbal or nutritional supplements. You may make copies of this form; keep an updated medication history and keep it along with your other health information records.

Name of medication	Date started	Date stopped/reason	Dose	Name of the health-care provider	Reason for taking	Side effects (if any)
Example: Lisinopril	1/1/2011		1 tablet once a day	Dr. Smith	High blood pressure	none

Lab Tests Record

This form may be used to monitor your CD4 cell count and viral load. There are extra columns to record any other lab tests or even your weight if you need to lose or gain weight. You may make copies of this form to track your lab test results and keep it along with your other health information records.

Date	CD4 cell count	Viral load			
Example: 1/1/2011	488	<20 copies			

Screening Tests for Women

Check the guidelines listed here to find out about important screening tests for women. The U.S. Preventive Services Task Force recommends these guidelines. Keep in mind that these are guidelines only. Your doctor or nurse will personalize the timing of the screening tests that you need based on many factors. Ask your doctor or nurse if you do not understand why a certain test is recommended for you. Check with your insurance plan to find out which tests are covered.

Screening tests	18 to 39 years	40 to 49 years	50 to 64 years	65 years and older
Blood pressure test	Get tested at least every 2 years if you have normal blood pressure (lower than 120/80). Get tested once a year if you have blood pressure between 120/80 and 139/89. Discuss treatment with your doctor or nurse if you have blood pressure 140/90 or higher.	Get tested at least every 2 years if you have normal blood pressure (lower than 120/80). Get tested once a year if you have blood pressure between 120/80 and 139/89. Discuss treatment with your doctor or nurse if you have blood pressure 140/90 or higher.	Get tested at least every 2 years if you have normal blood pressure (lower than 120/80). Get tested once a year if you have blood pressure between 120/80 and 139/89. Discuss treatment with your doctor or nurse if you have blood pressure 140/90 or higher.	Get tested at least every 2 years if you have normal blood pressure (lower than 120/80). Get tested once a year if you have blood pressure between 120/80 and 139/89. Discuss treatment with your doctor or nurse if you have blood pressure 140/90 or higher.
Bone mineral density test (osteoporosis screening)			Discuss with your doctor or nurse if you are at risk of osteoporosis.	Get tested at least once. Talk to your doctor or nurse about repeat testing.

(continued)

(continued)

Screening tests	18 to 39 years	40 to 49 years	50 to 64 years	65 years and older
Breast cancer screening (mammogram)		Discuss with your doctor or nurse.	Starting at the age of 50, get screened every 2 years.	Get screened every 2 years through age 74. At age 75 and older, ask your doctor or nurse if you need to be screened.
Cervical cancer screening (Pap test)	Get a Pap test at least every 3 years if you are 21 or older, or are younger than 21 and have been sexually active for at least 3 years.	Get a Pap test at least every 3 years.	Get a Pap test at least every 3 years.	Ask your doctor or nurse if you need to get a Pap test.
Chlamydia test	Get tested for chlamydia yearly through age 24 if you are sexually active or pregnant. Age 25 and older, get tested for chlamydia if you are at increased risk, pregnant or not pregnant.	Get tested for chlamydia if you are sexually active and at increased risk, pregnant or not pregnant.	Get tested for chlamydia if you are sexually active and at increased risk.	Get tested for chlamydia if you are sexually active and at increased risk.

Cholesterol test	Starting at the age of 20, get a cholesterol test regularly if you are at increased risk for heart disease. Ask your doctor or nurse how often you need your cholesterol tested.	Get a cholesterol test regularly if you are at increased risk for heart disease. Ask your doctor or nurse how often you need your cholesterol tested.	Get a cholesterol test regularly if you are at increased risk for heart disease. Ask your doctor or nurse how often you need your cholesterol tested.	Get a cholesterol test regularly if you are at increased risk for heart disease. Ask your doctor or nurse how often you need your cholesterol tested.
Colorectal cancer screening (using fecal occult blood testing, sigmoidoscopy, or colonoscopy)			Starting at the age of 50, get screened for colorectal cancer. Talk to your doctor or nurse about which screening test is best for you and how often you need it.	Get screened for colorectal cancer through age 75. Talk to your doctor or nurse about which screening test is best for you and how often you need it.
Diabetes screening	Get screened for diabetes if your blood pressure is higher than 135/80 or if you take medicine for high blood pressure.	Get screened for diabetes if your blood pressure is higher than 135/80 or if you take medicine for high blood pressure.	Get screened for diabetes if your blood pressure is higher than 135/80 or if you take medicine for high blood pressure.	Get screened for diabetes if your blood pressure is higher than 135/80 or if you take medicine for high blood pressure.

(continued)

(continued)

Screening tests	18 to 39 years	40 to 49 years	50 to 64 years	65 years and older
Gonorrhea test	Get tested for gonorrhea if you are sexually active and at increased risk, pregnant or not pregnant.	Get tested for gonorrhea if you are sexually active and at increased risk, pregnant or not pregnant.	Get tested for gonorrhea if you are sexually active and at increased risk.	Get tested for gonorrhea if you are sexually active and at increased risk.
HIV test	Get tested if you are at increased risk for HIV. Discuss your risk with your doctor or nurse. All pregnant women need to be tested for HIV.	Get tested if you are at increased risk for HIV. Discuss your risk with your doctor or nurse. All pregnant women need to be tested for HIV.	Get tested if you are at increased risk for HIV. Discuss your risk with your doctor or nurse.	Get tested if you are at increased risk for HIV. Discuss your risk with your doctor or nurse.
Syphilis test	Get tested for syphilis if you are at increased risk or pregnant.	Get tested for syphilis if you are at increased risk or pregnant.	Get tested for syphilis if you are at increased risk.	Get tested for syphilis if you are at increased risk.

Vaccines can protect you from harmful infections. Some adults think only children need vaccines, but this is not true. To find out what vaccines you may need, visit http://www.vaccines. gov, or the U.S. Department of Health and Human Services Office on Women's Health (http://www.womenshealth.gov; 800-994-9662; TDD: 888-220-5446).

Screening Tests for Men

Check the guidelines listed here to find out about important screening tests for men. The U.S. Preventive Services Task Force recommends these guidelines. Keep in mind that these are guidelines only. Your doctor or nurse will personalize the timing of the screening tests that you need based on many factors. Ask your doctor or nurse if you do not understand why a certain test is recommended for you. Check with your insurance plan to find out which tests are covered.

Screening tests	18 to 39 years	40 to 49 years	50 to 64 years	65 years and older
Abdominal aortic aneurysm screening				Get this one-time screening if you are between the age 65 and 75 and have ever smoked.
Blood pressure test	Get tested at least every 2 years if you have normal blood pressure (lower than 120/80). Get tested once a year if you have blood pressure between 120/80 and 139/89. Discuss treatment with your doctor or nurse if you have blood pressure 140/90 or higher.	Get tested at least every 2 years if you have normal blood pressure (lower than 120/80). Get tested once a year if you have blood pressure between 120/80 and 139/89. Discuss treatment with your doctor or nurse if you have blood pressure 140/90 or higher.	Get tested at least every 2 years if you have normal blood pressure (lower than 120/80). Get tested once a year if you have blood pressure between 120/80 and 139/89. Discuss treatment with your doctor or nurse if you have blood pressure 140/90 or higher.	Get tested at least every 2 years if you have normal blood pressure (lower than 120/80). Get tested once a year if you have blood pressure between 120/80 and 139/89. Discuss treatment with your doctor or nurse if you have blood pressure 140/90 or higher.

Cholesterol test	Starting at the age of 20 until 35, get a cholesterol test if you are at increased risk for heart disease. Starting at the age of 35 and older, get a cholesterol test regularly. Ask your doctor or nurse how often you need your cholesterol tested.	Get a cholesterol test regularly. Ask your doctor or nurse how often you need your cholesterol tested.	Get a cholesterol test regularly. Ask your doctor or nurse how often you need your cholesterol tested.	Get a cholesterol test regularly. Ask your doctor or nurse how often you need your cholesterol tested.
Colorectal cancer screening (using fecal occult blood testing, sigmoidoscopy, or colonoscopy)		Starting at age 50, get screened for colorectal cancer. Talk to your doctor or nurse about which screening test is best for you and how often you need it.		Get screened for colorectal cancer through age 75. Talk to your doctor or nurse about which screening test is best for you and how often you need it.

(continued)

(continued)

Screening tests	18 to 39 years	40 to 49 years	50 to 64 years	65 years and older
Diabetes screening	Get screened for diabetes if your blood pressure is higher than 135/80 or if you take medicine for high blood pressure.	Get screened for diabetes if your blood pressure is higher than 135/80 or if you take medicine for high blood pressure.	Get screened for diabetes if your blood pressure is higher than 135/80 or if you take medicine for high blood pressure.	Get screened for diabetes if your blood pressure is higher than 135/80 or if you take medicine for high blood pressure.
HIV test	Get tested if you are at increased risk for HIV. Discuss your risk with your doctor or nurse.	Get tested if you are at increased risk for HIV. Discuss your risk with your doctor or nurse.	Get tested if you are at increased risk for HIV. Discuss your risk with your doctor or nurse.	Get tested if you are at increased risk for HIV. Discuss your risk with your doctor or nurse.
Syphilis screening	Get tested for syphilis if you are at increased risk.	Get tested for syphilis if you are at increased risk.	Get tested for syphilis if you are at increased risk.	Get tested for syphilis if you are at increased risk.

Vaccines

Vaccines can protect you from harmful infections. Some adults think only children need vaccines, but this is not true. To find out what vaccines you may need, visit http://www.vaccines.gov.

The Gift of Health

You can never have enough information about how to prevent diseases and maintain your health. Our health is a gift, and something that we sometimes take for granted until a threat, like HIV, comes along. The best thing you can do for your health is to acquire the knowledge and skills needed to enhance, protect, and maintain it. So, even if some of the information in this book sounds repetitious, it is because it is so very important. Read on!

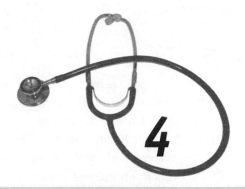

4

Lifestyle Changes and Healthy Habits

My dad died from a heart attack when he was 52. I thought I was doing pretty good keeping myself healthy. After I was diagnosed with HIV and the doctor was talking to me about my health, I discovered that I was doing things that put me at risk of having a heart attack just like my dad. It wasn't easy, but I gave up smoking 4 years ago.   PAUL, AGE 39

Everywhere you look these days you see countless ads for eating better, exercising more, and all the gimmicks that can make your life easier and healthier. But health is not easy to define. Many people seem to be able to maintain a healthy weight without any difficulty or getting up every morning and running 5 miles. But some of us struggle to lose a few pounds, do not sleep well at night, and are tired and stressed. Sitting on the couch, eating chips, and watching those ads is all we get done at the end of the day. Maybe there is a little bit of guilt about how we live, and we make a pledge to start eating better and exercising more on Monday, on the first of the month, on New Year's Day, or sometime in the future. But now that you know that you have a chronic health condition, it is more important than ever that you take care of yourself and do everything that you can to improve and maintain your health.

Many people kick off with a new health routine, such as starting an exercise regimen, and quit within a week. They are all gung ho the first couple of days and get up at 5:00 a.m. to walk or go to a gym, but then they have an early morning work meeting, they oversleep, or they have muscle aches from all the exercising. They tell themselves that they just do not have time to exercise. Or they just need to rest and wait awhile to restart. They overdo it at the beginning and find it easy to make excuses and stop before they have really even begun.

What Nurses Know...

There are many lifestyle choices and changes you can make that will improve your health, but you should consider a few words of advice before starting: Taking baby steps when making one or more lifestyle changes will ensure a greater chance of success.

The first step is to identify a goal. Many of us have so many goals, and we become stressed just thinking about making changes. So pick just one goal. Say you want to lose 10 pounds. Think about your life and your daily routine. What small changes can you make that will allow you to lose those 10 pounds? Keeping a food diary for a week or so will help you identify what your food habits are. Maybe you drink 2 liters of soda a day or eat ice cream at night. Perhaps you eat junk food when you are bored or stressed. Many times we are not even aware of how much we

eat or that we eat without even being hungry. Would it be possible to only drink 1 liter of soda a day and replace the other liter
with water? Or, switch to diet soda? These are simple ways to
begin making changes to your diet without feeling deprived or
stressed.

To reach that weight loss goal, you will also need to look at
your usual daily activity. Do you work an 8-hour job or are you a
stay-at-home mom? What ways could you add more activity into
your daily routine? There are many small ways to do that. You
could park a block away from workplace and walk one block to
and from your workplace every day. Maybe you could find time
to take an evening walk with your partner or neighbor. Just getting up 10 minutes earlier than usual to stretch is a great way to
start taking baby steps to achieve your goal of losing 10 pounds.
Once you have achieved success by reaching that goal, you will
feel more motivated and comfortable to make other goals that
will improve your health.

Nutrition and Exercise

Years ago, people with HIV often lost a great deal of weight
and muscle mass from advanced HIV disease or opportunistic infections. They also lost weight due to medication side
effects, which could cause nausea, vomiting, and diarrhea.
They were encouraged to eat foods loaded with fat, such as
ice cream and creamed soups, to maintain and increase their
weight. My, how times have changed! You will read more about
the history of HIV treatment and antiretroviral (ARV) medications in Chapter 5.

With newer medications and therapies, we rarely see persons
living with HIV who experience the severe weight loss that was
seen with this disease 15 or more years ago. However, we do know
that living with HIV and taking ARV medications may put you at
additional risk for heart disease, diabetes, and some cancers. For

those reasons, it is more important than ever for a person living with HIV to eat a nutritious healthy diet, exercise in moderation, and maintain a normal weight.

The U.S. Department of Agriculture gives guidelines to follow regarding the recommended servings of fruits, vegetables, grains, protein, and dairy. Trying to follow these guidelines will provide you with a diet lower in fat and higher in the nutrients needed to maintain health. Their Web site (www.myplate.gov) gives good information about each food category, and tips for successfully following their recommendations.

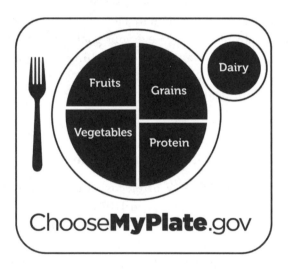

The following are some of the suggestions for maintaining a healthy and safe diet. If you have other health concerns, such as diabetes, talk to your provider about the diet you should be following. You can also ask your provider if it is advisable for you to talk to a dietitian about your diet and nutritional concerns. At the end of this book are some additional Web sites where you can find more information.

Tips for maintaining a healthy diet

○ Let the My Plate diagram (p. 54) guide your food choices and serving sizes
○ Choose a variety of fruits and vegetables to encourage you to eat a lower fat diet
○ Choose a diet that is low in saturated fat and cholesterol
○ Read food labels. Be aware of how much sodium and sugar are in processed foods and choose wisely
○ Limit the amount of salt you add to foods when cooking or eating
○ Limit the amount of alcohol you drink
○ Drink 8 to 10 cups of water daily
○ Practice food safety

Tips for best practices when shopping or cooking

○ Make a grocery list before you go to the store. This list will help keep you on track and hopefully avoid impulse buying. Beware of the chip aisle!
○ Eat a meal or snack before you shop. It is always tempting to buy more food than you need, and make less healthy food choices, when you are hungry
○ Read and compare labels. The first ingredient listed on the label means that it is the largest quantity item in the container. Also, compare different products. Low fat or sugar free does *not* mean low calorie
○ Choose fresh or frozen fruits and vegetables whenever possible. Canned items may be much higher in sodium. If you do buy canned foods, rinsing (if possible) will remove some of the salt before cooking or eating

○ Broil, bake, or boil foods instead of frying. You can also limit fat by using nonstick cooking sprays, trimming fat from meats, and removing skin from chicken or turkey

○ Try to limit salt you add to foods. Use herbs or seasonings for extra flavor

○ Save the pies, cakes, and ice cream for special treats. If you have a sweet tooth and need a dessert, choose fresh fruit or a low-fat dessert, such as angel food cake

Tips to reduce fat in your diet

○ Know the difference between the three types of fats and use *good* fats whenever possible

1. Saturated fats are found in lard, butter, meat's fat, dairy products made with whole milk, the skins of turkey and chicken, cocoa butter, and palm and coconut oil. These fats can *increase* your cholesterol levels and should be avoided whenever possible

2. Monounsaturated fats are found in olive, canola, and peanut oil and can *decrease* your cholesterol. These fats are good for you!

3. Polyunsaturated fats are found in oils from safflower, sunflower, soybean, corn, cottonseed, and sesame

○ Use dairy products that have low fat content. These include 1% or skim milk, low-fat yogurt, pudding or cottage cheese, mozzarella, ricotta, and parmesan cheeses

○ Eat whole grain breads and cereals. Even pastas are available in a whole grain version. Try something new like quinoa or barley. Potatoes that are baked or mashed are a good choice. Read the packaging on meat and choose lean meats, including chicken and turkey. Do not forget to remove the skin. Choose tuna that is canned in water rather than in oil

o Enjoy fresh, frozen, canned, or dried fruits and vegetables

o Eat or cook with fat-free vegetable soups or creamed soups made with skim milk

o Snack on nuts, carrot or celery sticks, unbuttered popcorn, pretzels, or plain crackers

o Indulge your sweet tooth with angel food cake, graham crackers, gingersnaps, or marshmallows

o Avoid fried or fatty meats including sausage, bacon, hot dogs, poultry with skin, and canned meats. Also, avoid gravies made from fat

o Avoid whole, 2%, or chocolate milk; cream; half and half; sour cream; cream cheese; and yogurt made with whole milk

o Avoid french fries, doughnuts, pastries, and biscuits

o Avoid butter, lard, and pork fat

Tips for food safety

o Keep your kitchen (refrigerator, stove, counters, floor, and sink) clean

o Always wash your hands before, during, and after preparing a meal. This is especially important if handling meat or poultry

o Clean cutting boards thoroughly after each use. Do not use cutting boards to cut up vegetables after using them for meat or poultry

o Wash all fruits and vegetables before using. A good rule of thumb is to wash them as soon as you bring them home and then again before you eat them

o Read food labels carefully and avoid buying foods after the "sell by" date

o Do not eat raw eggs or use raw eggs in health drinks

o Cook meat, poultry, and eggs thoroughly. No bloody or pink steak!
o Cook fish until it is flakey, not rubbery
o Do not eat raw meats or fish. If you really love sushi, talk to your provider if you can eat it in small quantities
o Refrigerate leftovers immediately; do not allow them to cool
o Do not keep leftovers more than 2 or 3 daysIf in doubt, throw it out!

Along with good nutrition, exercise is an important component of a healthy lifestyle. Research has found that exercise can help manage symptoms of metabolic syndrome. Reports estimate that up to 45% of people living with HIV may have metabolic syndrome, a condition that increases the risk of heart disease and diabetes.

Here are a few of the good reasons to make exercise a part of your health maintenance plan:

- Increases lean muscle mass
- Strengthens bones
- Increases strength and endurance
- Increases flexibility
- Increases energy levels
- Improves appetite
- Lowers triglycerides
- Helps control blood sugar
- Strengthens your heart
- Decreases belly fat
- Decreases stress
- Improves sleep

There are many ways to add more activity into your day, such as taking the stairs or getting up and walking around the house or the office every 1 or 2 hours. But to exercise to lose weight, you will need to devote more time to actual exercise.

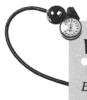

What Nurses Know...

Before beginning any exercise plan, you should discuss this with your healthcare provider. Discuss what types of exercise might be beneficial for you and if you need to take any precautions. Again, baby steps when starting this new goal.

Tips for starting an exercise plan

○ To make an exercise plan, you need to write down exactly what you want to accomplish. Do you want to lose weight? Gain more strength? Become more flexible? Then determine what types of exercise will best help you accomplish that goal

○ If you want to lose weight or gain muscle mass, now is the time to write down your measurements. You will want to write down how much you weigh and take measurements of your chest, abdomen, hips, upper arms, and thighs

○ It can be lonely and boring exercising alone. Ask a friend, family member, or neighbor to walk or work out with you

○ Remember it is all about taking baby steps. Start out slow, and do not overdo. Stop immediately if you become weak, dizzy, short of breath, or have chest pain

○ Depending on your health and ability, you may want to start out walking 30 minutes, three times a week and build up to walking 60 minutes, three to six times a week. If you are out of shape or fatigue easily, walk to the end of the driveway or the end of your block. Over time you will notice that you can walk further and without as much effort

○ You need to include a balanced diet with your exercise plan, and make sure to drink plenty of water. Dehydration and

low blood sugar can put a quick stop to your activity. You
need food for energy in order to succeed. Wait for 2 hours
after eating before you exercise. Drink water before, during,
and after your activities
o Do not exercise when you are feeling ill or fatigued

Different types of exercise will accomplish different goals.
Choose activities that you enjoy, like walking, biking, or swim-
ming. Consider trying something new like yoga or Tai Chi.
Below are some of the many exercise options for you to consider:

- **Aerobic exercise** is good for losing weight. It is also good
  for your heart because it raises your heart rate and makes it
  stronger. Types of aerobic exercise include fast walking, jog-
  ging, bicycling, and swimming
- **Resistance or strength-training exercises** improve muscle and
  bone strength. Types of resistance exercises include lifting
  weights, push-ups, and using equipment such as resistance
  bands or tubes. This type of exercise causes the muscles to contract. You should always allow the muscles to rest for a day or
  two between resistance exercises
- **Stretching and flexibility exercises** reduce stiffness and help the
  muscles perform better by increasing your flexibility, which in
  turn helps prevent injury. These exercises are done slowly and
  should not cause discomfort. They include stretching, either as
  part of warm up or cool down to aerobic exercises, or stretching on
  its own. Yoga is also another good exercise to promote flexibility

Smoking

If you smoke cigarettes or cigars, one of the best things you
could ever do for yourself is to stop! Easy to say, but it can be
so hard to do. Smoking does not make HIV worse, but it is well
known to cause cancer. If you smoke, you probably have more

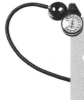

What Nurses Know...

You do not have to go to a gym in order to get a good work out. Walking is free, as is walking up and down stairs. You can buy resistance bands and weights, but you can also use different size cans of food you might have in your kitchen and use them as weights. Start out by lifting cans of soup and progress to large cans of tomatoes. You can also fill plastic milk cartons with water or sand to use as weights. Exercise does not have to be difficult or expensive.

secretions in your lungs than nonsmokers. These secretions make it easier for microorganisms to grow in your lungs and cause infection. People with HIV who smoke have a greater risk for having an AIDS-defining condition, such as pneumocystis pneumonia, or *Pneumocystis jiroveci* pneumonia, and also have more episodes of oral thrush. Smoking in general increases the risk of heart disease, high blood pressure, and stroke.

Tips on how to stop smoking

o Talk to your healthcare provider about your desire to stop smoking. Ask if any of the over-the-counter nicotine replacement therapies would be beneficial. Discuss if taking smoking cessation prescription medications (such as Zyban or Chantix) would be an option. Also discuss any side effects that could occur when taking these prescription medications

o Consider alternative therapies such as acupuncture or hypnotherapy

o If stress is the reason you smoke, find ways to reduce the factors that cause stress. If that is not possible, talk to your provider or case manager about support groups or counseling to help deal with stress

o If you have routines that trigger your need to smoke, like after finishing a meal, find an alternative way to use your hands or your time. Consider knitting or exercise as a way to combat the desire to smoke

o Ask friends and family members not to smoke when they are around you

It may not be easy, but it is possible to stop smoking. Take it one day at a time. Even cutting back one cigarette a day is a first step toward eliminating your unhealthy habit.

What Nurses Know...

Here's another reason not to smoke or to stop smoking: smoking makes skin look older and causes wrinkles!

Alcohol and Recreational Drugs

Alcohol (such as wine, beer, and liquor) and recreational drugs (such as cocaine, marijuana, and methamphetamines) can be dangerous for the person infected with HIV. They are known to lower your resistance to infection by causing blood abnormalities, interfere with your medications, and cause nutritional imbalances and deficiencies. There are also alcohol-related illnesses such as pancreatitis that may further impair your health and make it difficult to take your HIV medications. Using aspirin, ibuprofen, or other nonsteroidal drugs along with alcohol can cause stomach irritation (loss of appetite, nausea, vomiting) and stomach bleeding.

Alcohol and recreational drugs can cause loss of memory, confusion, hallucinations, delusions, depression, and difficulty sleeping. They are also associated with heart disease and liver disease. Because they are known to cause memory lapses or confusion, this could impair your ability to make good decisions, such as using condoms. Being under the influence of alcohol and recreation drugs puts you at risk for acquiring other sexually transmitted diseases. Dealing with alcohol and recreational drugs will be discussed in more detail later in this book.

Eliminating and/or Reducing Stress

Stress is so much a part of our life that many times we do not even recognize the damage it is causing to our physical and mental health. Negative impact of stress can lead to coronary artery (heart) disease, respiratory disorders, depression, alcoholism, and even suicide. How many times do you get a stress-induced headache? Or, feel the muscles of your shoulders or back tightening? How many times have you heard someone say they were too stressed to eat or sleep? Stress affects everyone and it affects how we care for ourselves and live healthfully.

Here are some steps you can take to reduce your stress:

- **Identify the cause of your stress.** Are you worried about taking medication? Worried about paying your bills? Write down what you feel is the cause of your stress. Then write down ideas of what you might be able to do to change or reduce the stress. If you are worried about taking medication, is it possible to ask your pharmacist if they can talk to you about your concerns?
- **Make a list of your priorities and brainstorm how to accomplish them**. If taking HIV medications is a high priority, identify any obstacles you might encounter in taking them. Do you often get up late and run out the door? Do you fall asleep in front of the TV every night and stumble to bed? List ways that you will always have your medications in a convenient location, ready to take. Do you need a pill box/organizer or another way to remember? Talk to your pharmacist, case manager, or peer

educator about ways to successfully take your medications. Take each priority and process it this way

- **Seek professional help.** If you are experiencing depression or severe anxiety, seek the help of a professional. Talk to your provider about your depression or anxiety. Your provider may be able to treat your depression or may want you to see a mental health professional to get it under control
- **Join a support group.** Talk to your case manager or peer educator about local support groups. There may also be local community educational programs about living with HIV that you can attend. Talking to other people who are experiencing similar situations may help you see things in a different light
- **Exercise or do an activity you enjoy.** Sometimes you can ease the stress by exercising or doing another activity like listening to music. Call a friend you have not heard from for a while. Both of you may benefit from the time you spend talking to each other

Remember, you are not alone. Allow your friends and family the opportunity to help. Talk to your provider or case manager about other alternatives to dealing with your stress.

Alternative or Complementary Medicine

Alternative or complementary medicine is any healing practice that is not within the realm of "mainstream" medicine. Many practitioners of complementary medicine focus on healing the whole person and promote self-care and self-healing. Some alternative therapies may be based on cultural or historical rituals. Some therapies may be very similar to traditional medicine such as good nutrition, while others may be based on folk knowledge. Many aspects of alternative medicine have not been researched and do not have scientific evidence to back up their claims.

One thing to remember if you are considering an alternative therapy is that alternative medicines do not treat HIV. There is no magical herb that will cure HIV. In fact, many herbs may interfere with antiretrovirals. One such herb is St. John's wort. This herb is sometimes taken to relieve mild depression. When taken with the protease inhibitor, Crixivan, it decreases the amount of Crixivan in the blood, which could lead to drug resistance. Garlic supplements can also reduce the blood levels of another protease inhibitor, saquinavir. There are many herbs and supplements that have not been studied enough to know what their effect will be on HIV or how they interact with ARVs. If you would like to take an alternative therapy, such as an herb or supplement, please discuss with your provider before doing so.

We have discussed some other activities earlier in this chapter that are sometimes considered *alternative*. These include yoga, meditation, or massage. All of these may help you relax and reduce your stress.

Healthy Habits

HAND WASHING

More and more people are becoming aware of the need to practice good hand washing. You will see wall dispensers of hand sanitizer in hallways of hospitals, outside elevators, and in places where large numbers of people congregate, such as airports or sports stadiums. For a person infected with HIV, hand washing is one of the most important health habits they can practice to prevent getting ill from an infection or passing on germs.

WHEN TO WASH YOUR HANDS

- Before, during, and after preparing food
- Before you eat
- After using the toilet
- After changing diapers or cleaning up a child who has used the toilet
- After coughing, sneezing, or blowing your nose
- After cleaning any wounds, cuts or scrapes, or changing dressings
- After caring for someone who is ill
- After touching animals, cleaning cages, or picking up feces
- After touching garbage or working in dirt, including potting soil used for houseplants

THE CORRECT WAY TO WASH YOUR HANDS

- Wet your hands with clean running water and apply a small amount of liquid or bar soap. It does not matter if the water is warm or cold
- Make a lather by rubbing your hands together
- Scrub all areas of your hands, including the backs of your hands and between fingers, and as much under your nails as possible
- Rub/scrub your hands for at least 20 seconds continuously
- Rinse your hands with clean water
- Dry your hands with a clean cloth or allow to air dry
- *If you do not have soap and water, you can use a hand sanitizer that contains at least 60% alcohol. But keep in mind that hand sanitizers do not kill all types of germs and are not effective if hands are visibly dirty*

You should also encourage people you live with or who visit you to wash their hands.

TAKING CARE OF YOUR SKIN

People with HIV may experience occasional problems with their skin. They may notice rashes, itch, red bumps, dry patches, or dark or purple-colored lesions. These may be minor annoyances or be a symptom that should be reported to your provider. It is important that you be aware of what is normal and not normal for you. Maybe you always have dry skin in the winter or develop a rash when you use a certain soap; but when you notice changes in your skin and do not have an explanation, you will need to decide if it is something that should be reported to your provider.

If you develop a rash after starting a new medication, it is a good idea to call the clinic or office and report it to the staff. You may be told to take an antihistamine, such as Benadryl. If the rash worsens, you will most likely be told to discontinue the medication. The provider will need your information to weigh the options and determine if there is another medication that can be substituted.

SKIN CARE

Protect your skin from the sun (remember too much sun causes wrinkles)

1. Limit your time outside when the sun's rays are the strongest, 10:00 a.m. to 4:00 p.m.
2. Wear long-sleeved shirts and other protective clothing, including hats
3. Apply sunscreen 30 minutes before going outdoors and reapply every 2 hours

Some people with HIV may also have a tendency to develop *folliculitis,* or infection of the hair follicle. Symptoms include itching, a red rash, or pus-filled lesions. While it can occur anywhere there is hair, folliculitis most typically develops

- On the face or scalp
- On the chest or back
- Under the arms
- On the legs

The causes of folliculitis include

- Shaving
- Rubbing from clothes that are too tight
- Clogging of pores by dirt and oils

Prevention of folliculitis

- Using an electric shaver rather than a razor
- Avoiding clothing that is too tight or rubs against certain areas of the body prone to folliculitis
- Keeping skin clean and dry
- Depending on the type of infection, your provider may prescribe oral antibiotics, antibiotic creams, shampoo, or antifungal cream

Seborrheic Dermatitis

This is the most common skin problem experienced by people living with HIV. While it only occurs in about 5% of the general population, it occurs in up to 90% of people with advanced HIV disease. While the cause is not entirely known, it is thought to be due to an excess of skin oil and a yeast called malassezia.

Other risk factors for seborrheic dermatitis include

- May run in families
- Stress
- Fatigue
- Weather extremes
- Oily skin
- Infrequent shampooing or cleaning of the skin
- Lotions or skin care products containing alcohol
- Obesity
- Other skin conditions, such as acne

Symptoms

- White to yellowish flaky scales over pink patches of skin
- May be itchy
- Forms usually where skin is oily
- Most common areas are scalp, eyelids and eyebrows, behind the ears, creases of the nose, beard, mid-chest, back, underarms, and groin
- Hair loss

Treatment

- Over-the-counter dandruff or medicated shampoos
- Antifungal creams, such as ketoconazole (requires prescription)
- Corticosteroid creams, such as hydrocortisone
- Antiretrovirals (HIV medications), if indicated

• Even with treatment, seborrheic dermatitis may reoccur. Be certain to discuss reoccurrences with your provider and ask for refills on any prescription creams so that you will have them available if it does reoccur

While we have discussed a couple of common skin conditions, it is important to recognize that skin provides an important layer of protection against infection. Avoiding infections is important for people living with HIV. Many times, skin is damaged by years of exposure to the sun. Now is the time to begin giving your skin the care and protection it needs and deserves. Treat your skin gently by doing the following steps:

1. Limit your time soaking in a hot bath or taking a hot shower. Hot water strips oils from the skin. Use warm water when bathing to retain those oils
2. Use a liquid soap, which is usually less harsh on the skin. Soaps containing a moisturizer may also help relieve dry skin
3. Apply body lotions or creams while skin is still damp from bathing or showering, which helps improve dry skin
4. Use skin care lotions and creams that are fragrance free
5. A cool lotion kept in the refrigerator may be soothing to itchy skin
6. Add moisture to the air. During winter, air can become dry, so use a humidifier or heat a pot of water until you see steam and keep at a low temperature to add humidity
7. When shaving, face or legs, use a lotion or shaving cream to protect your skin

A healthy diet can also help your skin.

1. Research suggests that a diet rich in vitamin C and low in carbohydrates and fats may improve your skin
2. Eat a diet that contains veggies, whole grains, and lean proteins

What Nurses Know...

Remember not to share razors. They may be contaminated with small amounts of blood. Change your own personal razor often because used razors can also house bacteria, and using an old razor can lead to infections. The same goes for toothbrushes too!

DENTAL/ORAL CARE

Mouth infections are common in people with HIV. Sometimes, dentists will recommend to their clients that they get an HIV test because of certain conditions they see in the mouth. If your immune system is impaired, it can be difficult for it to control infections, including those that can occur in your mouth. To take good care of your mouth and maintain your health, we recommend you do the following:

- Brush your teeth and gums at least twice a day, especially after meals and at bedtime
- Use a soft-bristled toothbrush to avoid bleeding of gums
- Floss between teeth at least once a day, unless gums are tender or bleed easily
- Never share toothbrushes or other devices used to clean teeth such as a Waterpik or a toothpick. They might contain small amounts of blood that could transmit HIV
- Check the inside of your mouth every day. This also includes your lips, teeth, gums, tongue, and roof of your mouth. Notify your healthcare team if you notice any changes
- Report to your healthcare team if you find the following changes:

  1. Red patches
  2. White patches
  3. Open sores

4. Difficulty swallowing
5. Sore mouth, especially when you eat or drink
6. Swelling or lumps. With your eyes closed, feel both sides of your face and your neck. Notice if you feel any swelling or lumps. Contact your provider if the swelling or lumps do not go away in a week or if they become painful. If you are ever uncertain about what you are feeling or seeing, do not hesitate to contact a member of your healthcare team for advice
7. Make and keep appointment with your dentist every 6 months to have your teeth and gums examined and your teeth cleaned. Gum disease (gingivitis) is a common condition experienced by people living with HIV. To prevent tooth and bone loss, gingivitis needs to be treated by a dentist as soon as possible

What Nurses Know...

Your dentist is a member of your healthcare team and should be told that you have HIV. Having that information will allow your dentist to better inform you of symptoms to watch for and report to your provider.

If you do get a mouth infection or irritation, here are some comfort measures to sooth a sore mouth:

- Avoid salty, spicy, or acidic foods
- Avoid using mouthwashes containing alcohol, which can dry and irritate the inside of your mouth
- If your gums are too sore to use a toothbrush, wipe your teeth, tongue, and inside of your cheeks with gauze pads moistened with warm water
- Rinse your mouth three to four times a day with warm salt water (1/4 teaspoon salt to 1/2 glass of warm water)
- Eat cold, smooth foods that will help sooth a sore mouth, such as Popsicles, Jell-O, or sherbet, and drink cold liquids

Keeping Your Environment Clean and Safe

Living in a clean environment is important for someone who is protecting their immune system from unwanted germs. Most of it is just plain common sense, but here are some safe habits you should practice to protect yourself and others:

- Clean your bathroom weekly. Clean shower stalls with a solution of one cup bleach to one gallon water
- Clean around and under appliances, such as refrigerators and stoves, where molds and fungi may grow
- Clean the inside of your refrigerator and toss out outdated foods and leftovers as necessary
- Wash dishes as usual. There is no need for separate dishes
- Do not let water stand in humidifiers or vaporizers. Clean weekly to avoid growth of molds or fungi
- Use separate cloths to clean the countertops and the sink and a separate cloth for the floor
- Bandages or feminine hygiene products should be double-bagged when put in the garbage

Accidents May Happen

You may accidentally cut yourself, become ill and vomit, or have diarrhea. These things happen. Your family or friends, or even strangers, might want to help. It is important that they do not come in direct contact with your blood or body fluids (urine, feces, vomit, and semen) if such accidents should occur. Always keep a pair of latex gloves available for such an incident. If blood or vomit needs to be cleaned up from a countertop or floor, the area should be wiped up with hot, soapy water and then disinfected with a bleach solution of one cup bleach to one gallon water. If you are in a serious accident and an ambulance is called, remember to tell the emergency medical technician or paramedic that you have HIV disease.

Pets

A pet is an important member of the family. Pets give unconditional love and often know when you are happy, sad, or stressed. Playing with your pet can reduce stress and may increase your activity, such as when you walk your dog.

It is not possible for you to give your pet HIV, but it is possible for your pet to pass on infections. Here are a few safety precautions to take when caring for your pet:

- Always wash your hands with soap and water after playing with or caring for your pets
- Pets can pass on infections, especially through contact with their feces. When picking up poop or cleaning cages, you should wear rubber gloves, and wash your hands as soon as you remove the gloves
- Change litter boxes every day. If at all possible, get someone else to do that for you
- Be careful of what your pet eats and drinks. Do not let them drink from the toilet, eat raw or undercooked meat, or food from the garbage. Do not let them eat the feces on the ground from other dogs or cats
- Avoid pets that are ill, especially if they have diarrhea. Ask a friend or family to care for them
- Do not pet stray animals; they could scratch or bite you
- If you are scratched or bitten by your pet or a stray animal, wash the wound immediately with soap and water. Seek medical attention if the scratch or bitten part becomes red and painful or has pus, or if you develop a fever
- Do not handle reptiles such as snakes, lizards, or turtles. If you do handle them, wash your hands immediately with warm, soapy water

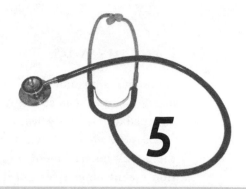

5

Antiretroviral Medications

You don't have to worry about me, I'm going to learn all I can about HIV treatment, and I promise to take these ARV medications faithfully every day for the rest of my life. I want to live! CELIA, NEWLY DIAGNOSED WITH HIV AT AGE 56

A Little History about HIV Treatment

Today, 30 years into the HIV epidemic, a person who is diagnosed early in the course of HIV disease can expect to live a normal life span and enjoy good health if he/she has access to healthcare and to treatment with antiretroviral (ARV) medications. ARV treatment must be taken every day for a lifetime and consists of taking a combination of medications (usually one to three pills) faithfully without missing doses and without interrupting therapy. However, the treatment of HIV disease with ARV medications has not always been this simple and the prognosis has not always been so bright. The treatment of HIV disease has changed dramatically over time.

In 1981, when HIV was first recognized in the United States, there was no treatment and being diagnosed with HIV infection meant almost certain death. In 1987, the first ARV medication, azidothymidine (AZT) or zidovudine, became widely available. Taking AZT back in the 1980s meant setting an alarm and taking high doses of AZT around the clock every few hours. Unfortunately, it soon became clear that treating HIV with just one medication was not effective and HIV could not be controlled in this manner.

A landmark breakthrough in the treatment of HIV came in the 1990s with the realization that a combination of ARV medications was needed to effectively treat the disease. In 1996, when a new class of HIV medication called protease inhibitors (PIs) became available, HIV suddenly changed from a death sentence to a disease that could be chronic and manageable.

Although combination ARV treatment was helping people with HIV to live longer, the ARV medications of the late 1990s were sometimes pretty difficult to take. It required that people take handfuls of pills several times a day. Not only did people have to take a lot of pills, but also many of these ARV medication combinations caused unpleasant side effects and some had life-threatening toxicities. Many people had difficulty taking their ARV medications faithfully and would skip doses or even stop treatment, which often led to HIV drug resistance and treatment failure. In addition, we did not know as much back then about how to sequence ARV medications and some of the medications were not potent enough, so sometimes people with HIV would develop HIV drug resistance, even if they took their ARV medications perfectly as prescribed.

In the 2000s, new formulations and classes of ARV medications became available that were more "user friendly" and more potent. These advances meant less pills, less side effects, and once-daily dosing. In addition, combined HIV medications also became available, making HIV treatment with a single pill per day a reality (i.e., one pill that contains three ARV medications). Treatment for HIV with ARV medications has come a long way, from taking handfuls of pills two or three times a day to now, when most of the patients take only one to four pills once a day.

ARV Medications

The medications used to treat HIV infection are called ARVs. There are several categories of ARV medications, and they will be discussed in detail in this chapter. ARVs must be used in combination. The successful treatment of HIV disease depends on prescribing an effective combination of ARVs and ensuring that the individual who is living with HIV takes his/her ARV medications faithfully, every day, for the rest of his/her life. ARV medications suppress HIV viral load by interrupting with the HIV life cycle, which means that HIV cannot replicate (make copies of itself) and therefore cannot damage the immune system. Shutting down HIV replication with ARV medications also allows the immune system to rebuild itself and allows the CD4 cell count to increase. While there is no cure for HIV infection, treatment with ARV medications allows HIV to be a chronic disease that can be successfully managed for a lifetime.

There are several categories of ARV medications available to treat HIV disease. All ARVs interrupt the HIV life cycle, preventing HIV from replicating. You can refer to the diagram of the HIV life cycle in Chapter 1. ARVs are used in combination and do not work if they are given as monotherapy (just one medication). Typically, three ARVs must be taken together for successful treatment of HIV disease. Fortunately, there are a number of ARVs available and several combinations of ARVs that are very effective for the treatment of HIV disease. HIV treatment regimens must be individualized, and several factors need to be taken into consideration when choosing a combination of ARV medications. Factors include things such as other health problems and other medications an individual is taking. In addition, the order in which ARVs are prescribed is also critical, particularly among individuals who have some degree of HIV drug resistance. There is more information about HIV drug resistance later in this chapter.

What Nurses Know...

It is important to have your ARV medications prescribed by a healthcare provider who has plenty of experience treating HIV disease, or who has ready access to experts in the field who can help make decisions about ARV therapy choices. Several research studies have shown that, in general, when experienced HIV healthcare providers treat people with HIV disease, they have better health outcomes.

NUCLEOSIDE REVERSE TRANSCRIPTASE INHIBITORS

Nucleoside reverse transcriptase inhibitors (NRTIs) are a category of ARV medications that interrupt the HIV life cycle by stopping the DNA chain. NRTIs act early in the HIV life cycle and are incorporated in the newly created DNA strand causing the chemical reaction, and replication, to end. Here are the currently available NRTIs.

Zidovudine (also called AZT and ZDV, Retrovir) was the first ARV medication to be approved by the Food and Drug Administration (FDA) in the United States for the treatment of HIV infection. Zidovudine is still widely used, especially for the treatment of HIV-infected pregnant women to prevent mother-to-infant HIV transmission. Zidovudine is also used to treat infants born to HIV-infected mothers for the first 6 weeks of life to further help prevent the infant from seroconverting and becoming HIV infected.

Didanosine (also called DDI, Videx) was the second ARV medication to be approved by the FDA in the United States for the treatment of HIV infection. Didanosine is not widely used in the United States today, primarily due to the development of newer ARV medications that have less side effects and toxicities than didanosine.

Zalcitabine (also called ddC, Hivid) was an early ARV medication. It is no longer used as newer ARV medications with less toxicities have been developed. This ARV has been discontinued by the manufacturer.

Stavudine (also called d4T, Zerit) was an early nonnucleoside reverse transcriptase inhibitors (NNRTI). Stavudine is not widely used in the United States today due to the development of newer ARV medications that have less side effects and toxicities than stavudine.

Lamivudine (also called 3TC, Epivir) is approved for the treatment of both HIV and hepatitis B. Lamivudine is available as a single agent or in combination pills (pills to treat HIV that contain more than one ARV).

Abacavir (also called ABC, Ziagen) is available as a single agent, in combination with lamivudine (Epzicom), or in combination with zidovudine and lamivudine (Trizivir). Before starting abacavir, you should have a lab test called HLA B5701 to determine if you are allergic to the ARV. Although only a very small number of people will be allergic to this medication, the allergy can be life threatening, so it is very important to have the lab test before starting abacavir.

Emtricitabine (also called FTC, Emtriva) is similar in action to lamivudine; it is used for treatment of HIV and hepatitis B. Emtricitabine is available as a single agent or in combination with tenofovir (Viread).

NUCLEOTIDE ANALOG REVERSE-TRANSCRIPTASE INHIBITORS

Normally, nucleoside analogs are converted into nucleotide analogs by the body. This type of drug skips those conversion steps.

There is one such drug that is approved and used to treat HIV today, tenofovir.

Tenofovir (also known as tenofovir disoproxil fumarate, brand trade name Viread) is a nucleotide analog that is approved for the treatment of both HIV and hepatitis B. It is available as a single agent or in combination with emtricitabine (emtriva).

NONNUCLEOSIDE REVERSE-TRANSCRIPTASE INHIBITORS

NNRTIs are a category of ARV medications that are similar to the nucleotide and nucleoside reverse transcriptase inhibitors as they interrupt the HIV life cycle at the same place, but NNRTIs have a slightly different way in which they work.

Efavirenz (also known as EFV, Sustiva) is available as a single agent or in combination with tenofovir and emtricitabine (Atripla).

Nevirapine (Viramune) is used in combination with other ARVs for the treatment of HIV disease and has also been used as a single agent for the prevention of transmission of HIV from mother to baby, particularly in developing countries.

Delavirdine (Rescriptor) is an NNRTI that is rarely used due to the development of newer NNRTIs with more potency.

Etravirine (Intelence) is a newer NNRTI that was approved by the FDA in 2008. Etravirine has a resistance pattern different from that of the older NNRTIs (efavirenz and nevirapine), so it can be used in people who have become resistant to the older NNRTIs.

Rilpivirine (Edurant) is the newest NNRTI and was approved by the FDA in May 2011. Rilpivirine also has a drug resistance pattern different from that of the older NNRTIs. It is touted as the smallest ARV pill and is available as a single agent or as a combination pill with tenofovir and emtricitabine (Complera).

PROTEASE INHIBITORS

PIs are a class of drugs used to treat HIV and hepatitis C. In the treatment of HIV, PIs stop the HIV life cycle by inhibiting the activity of protease, an enzyme that HIV uses at the end of the life cycle to assemble new viral particles. PIs were the second class of ARV drugs developed and their development resulted in a landmark change: the ability to treat HIV disease for a lifetime and change it from a fatal to a chronic disease.

Saquinavir (Fortovase, Invirase) was the first PI approved by the FDA and is rarely used today.

Ritonavir (Norvir) was originally released as a single agent but has made its mark in HIV treatment as a "booster." In other words, ritonavir is now widely used in lower doses in combination with other PIs to increase their effectiveness.

Indinavir (Crixivan) was an early PI and played a significant role in transforming HIV from a fatal to a chronic disease. It is not used as much today due to the availability of newer more potent PIs with less side effects and/or once-daily dosing.

Nelfinavir (Viracept) was an early PI and played a significant role in preventing mother to baby transmission of HIV. It is dosed twice daily, so it is not as popular as some of the newer once-daily dosed PIs. It is still used in the treatment of HIV-infected pregnant women, especially in developing countries.

Fosamprenavir (Lexiva) can be given once daily when used by individuals who have not been treated with PIs in the past and who do not have drug resistance. For individuals who are ARV treatment experienced, fosamprenavir is given twice a day. Fosamprenavir must be given with ritonavir as a "booster."

Atazanavir (Reyataz) is a once-daily PI that must be given with ritonavir as a booster. Atazanavir cannot be taken with proton pump inhibitors (Prilosec, Protonix, Nexium, omeprazole) because these drugs lower the effectiveness of atazanavir. If taken with medications that reduce acid (Pepcid, Zantac, famotidine, ranitidine, TUMS, Maalox), then one must take atazanavir separately from these medications and the separation time should be 12 hours.

Darunavir (Prezista) is a PI that can be given once daily to individuals who have not had treatment with PIs in the past and twice daily to individuals who are treatment experienced. Both once-daily and twice-daily darunavir must be given with ritonavir as a booster.

Tipranavir (Aptivus) is a PI that is on the market but not utilized very often. It must be given with ritonavir as a booster.

INTEGRASE INHIBITORS

Integrase inhibitors are a fairly new class of drugs used to treat HIV. In the treatment of HIV, integrase inhibitors stop the HIV life cycle by the enzyme integrase, which is essential for HIV replication. The development of integrase inhibitors was critical for people who have significant drug resistance to the PIs and NNRTIs. The introduction of integrase inhibitors brought with it the ability to create viable treatment regimens for individuals who previously had limited HIV treatment options.

Raltegravir (Isentress) is currently the only integrase inhibitor on the market. It must be given in combination with other ARVs and it is dosed twice daily.

ENTRY INHIBITORS

Maraviroc (Selzentry) is a CCR5-receptor antagonist. This class of ARV was developed to address the challenge of effective treatment for individuals with HIV drug resistance. It is used in combination with other ARV medications and is typically reserved for use by individuals with HIV drug resistance. A person *must* have a laboratory test called a tropism (or trofile) test prior to starting maraviroc to ensure that the drug will be effective.

Enfuvirtide (also known as T-20 or Fuzeon) is the only ARV that is injected. A person taking this medication gives himself/herself a shot twice a day. T-20 was developed in response to the need for ARV that had effectiveness for individuals with HIV drug resistance. It is not widely used because newer effective ARVs for drug-resistant individuals have been developed. Also because it has to be injected, many individuals who need this class of ARV drug prefer maraviroc since it comes as a pill.

ONE-A-DAY TREATMENTS

There are two "one-a-day" treatments available to treat HIV disease. These treatment options consist of one pill that contains three ARV medications in it.

Atripla was the first complete treatment for HIV in one pill brought to the market in 2006. It is a combination pill that contains efavirenz, tenofovir, and emtricitabine and it is dosed once daily.

Complera was the second complete treatment for HIV in one combination pill, which contains rilpivirine, tenofovir, and emtricitabine. The FDA approved it in August of 2011.

Clinical Trials

There are usually ARVs "in the pipeline." These are new medications for the future that are still in experimental stages. As new ARVs are invented and become promising for treatment, they are studied in humans by means of scientific clinical trials. Such clinical trials typically occur in communities that have large universities, often referred to as AIDS Clinical Trial Groups. Clinical trials offer a way for people living with HIV to participate in research that may lead to better treatments in the future. For information about HIV clinical trials, visit http://www.aidsinfo.nih.gov/ClinicalTrials/Default.aspx.

Side Effects and Toxicities of ARV Medications

While many significant advances have been made in the treatment of HIV disease with ARV medications, there are still side effects and toxicities that can occur, and it is important for you to be familiar with them. Be sure to read the information that comes with your ARV medications from the pharmacy and to ask your healthcare provider for handouts that list information about how to take your ARV medications and what side effects to report. Many of the toxicities that can occur with ARV medications are usually detected early through laboratory monitoring.

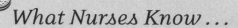

What Nurses Know...

It is important to get lab work done on a regular basis when you are taking ARV medications to catch toxicities early before they become a problem. It is also important to report to your healthcare provider any side effects or concerns about your ARV medications as soon as they start. Sometimes people wait too long to report side effects or concerns and this can result in problems that could have been avoided. Also, do not stop taking the ARV medications and wait until your next appointment to tell your healthcare provider because stopping the medications may contribute to drug resistance. Contact your healthcare provider and report the symptoms when they occur.

ALLERGIC REACTIONS

Any medication can produce an allergic reaction, and these reactions can vary from individual to individual. Common symptoms that can be associated with allergic reactions to ARV medications are rash, fever, redness of the skin, nausea, and vomiting. If you have any of these symptoms, or other concerns, you should contact your healthcare provider as soon as possible.

COMMON SIDE EFFECTS

Some of the ARV medications have side effects that are self-limiting; in other words, they disappear after you have been taking the medication for a period of time. But some side effects do not disappear and can interfere with quality of life. If you have any side effects or concerns with your ARV mediations, you should report them to your healthcare provider so that he/she can help you sort out if your side effects are temporary or if they need to be addressed. Common side effects of ARV medications include bloating, diarrhea, nausea, and mild headache. If you have rash, fever, vomiting, abdominal (belly) pain, dizziness, severe head-ache, or any other significant concerns, these are not common side effects and you should call your healthcare provider or go to the emergency room for evaluation.

POTENTIAL TOXICITIES OF ARV MEDICATIONS

ARV medications can cause serious problems (toxicities) like liver and kidney problems. Most of these toxicities can be detected early, before they become a problem, with monitoring of your lab work (blood and urine testing). At first, your healthcare provider will ask you to have more frequent lab work when you initially start a new regimen of ARV medications because seri-ous toxicities will usually occur early in the course of treatment. After you have been on the same ARV for a while, the frequency of lab monitoring will decrease to every 3 months and then every 6 months. It is very rare for a serious life-threatening toxicity to occur after a person has been on the same ARV regimen for a long period of time.

Metabolic complications. Some people develop metabolic problems—such as high blood pressure, high cholesterol, or type 2 diabetes—after being on ARV therapy. Sometimes it is difficult to determine if it is the ARV medications themselves that are causing the metabolic problems or if it is due to lifestyle factors or other risk factors like family history. Most of the time it is all of these things combined that can lead to metabolic problems among people who have HIV disease. Sometimes the ARV medi-cation regimen can be changed and this will help the metabolic problem. But the usual course of action is to treat the problem. For example, if you develop high blood pressure after you start taking ARV medications and your ARV medications are working well for your HIV, then most likely you will be advised to change your lifestyle (lose weight, reduce your salt intake, exercise). You might also be prescribed a medication for your blood pressure.

Body composition changes. Some of the ARV medications, especially some of the older ones that are no longer used, lead to changes in body fat distribution. For some people, fat redistributes and deposits in the abdomen, breasts, or neck. Another fat redistribution problem that has also been seen with ARV therapy is the loss of fat in the cheeks, arms, and legs. Sometimes changing the ARV regimen can help reverse this problem. Again, the newer ARV medications do not seem to have the degree of body composition problems that the older ARV medications of the 1990s did.

Bone health issues. Some ARV medications, especially PIs, can cause osteopenia (bone loss) and/or osteoporosis (soft bones). About 50% of people living with HIV who have been on HIV medicines for some time, especially PIs, have osteopenia/osteoporosis. Everyone with HIV who has been on ARV medications, especially PIs, should have a dual-energy x-ray absorptiometry (DEXA) (bone density) test. A DEXA test is not invasive and is not uncomfortable. There is treatment for osteopenia and for osteoporosis.

What Nurses Know...

Vitamin D and calcium deficiency can also increase the risk of osteoporosis. Most people are not at high risk for vitamin D deficiency (except teenage girls and postmenopausal women). If your vitamin D level is less than 20 IU, you should receive supplemental vitamin D (600 units daily). Because osteoporosis is common among women, many women take calcium with vitamin D and this type of vitamin supplement is enough. Men and women who are living with HIV should eat foods that are high in calcium and vitamin D and also take calcium and vitamin D supplements if needed.

IMMUNE RECONSTITUTION INFLAMMATORY SYNDROME

Immune reconstitution inflammatory syndrome (IRIS) is a serious health condition that can occur when ARV medications are started. Paradoxically, the improvement in the immune system can cause illness as a result of the body's aggressive inflammatory response to any previously unrecognized infections. IRIS is typically seen in people who have advanced HIV disease (AIDS) and who have an opportunistic infection that has not been recognized prior to starting the ARV medications. IRIS occurs most often in people who are newly diagnosed with HIV disease and who have a very low CD4 cell count (below 200) at the time of their diagnosis and then are started on ARV medications. If a person develops IRIS, hospitalization may be needed. While IRIS can be life threatening, usually the condition lasts about 2 months and resolves on its own with supportive measures.

Interactions between ARVs and Other Medications (Drug–Drug Interactions)

When someone has a chronic illness, like HIV, and has to take medications for a lifetime, there will likely come a time when other medications are also prescribed for other health problems that come up. All medications can have interactions with each other. Sometimes drugs that interact with each other have serious consequences. There are three common drug-drug interaction scenarios: (i) one drug can lower the effect of another drug; (ii) one drug can increase the level of another drug, making the dose too high; or (iii) one drug can counteract the effect of another drug, making it ineffective. Drug interactions can happen quite easily, and without you even knowing it. In addition to prescription drugs, herbs and supplements can also interact with ARVs. This information is discussed in Chapter 4 in the "Alternative or Complementary Medicine" section.

Here is a typical example of how a drug-drug interaction might happen.

Fred has been seeing Dr. Jones for HIV for 3 years. Fred is doing great with his HIV treatment and has a CD4 count of over 1,000 and an undetectable viral load. Fred is on his second regimen of HIV treatment because he had some HIV drug resistance in the past. Fred gets his ARV prescriptions filled at an HIV specialty pharmacy that is near Dr. Jones' office.

Fred goes to see Dr. Smith about some stomach issues he's having. Dr. Smith is a gastrointestinal specialist who practices at a different hospital than Dr. Jones, so he has no way to access Dr. Jones' medical records of Fred. Dr. Smith asks Fred "What medications are you taking?" and Fred tells him the names of his ARV medications. He can't remember the dosages, and he can't call the specialty pharmacy to check the dosages because it is Saturday and they are closed. He forgets to tell Dr. Smith about one of the ARVs he is taking.

Dr. Smith gives him a prescription, and he wants to start the medication right away, so he goes to the local 24-hour pharmacy (not the one where he gets his ARVs filled). Fred starts taking the medication for his stomach problem and the problem subsides. Two months later, he goes for his routine HIV checkup with Dr. Jones. He asks, "Are you taking any new medications?" and he pulls out the bottle with the new prescription medication from Dr. Smith. Well, Dr. Jones gets a very concerned look on his face because it turns out that the ARV medication Fred forgot to tell Dr. Smith about has a drug-drug interaction with the new medication that he prescribed for his stomach. The medication that Fred is taking for his stomach problem lowers the level of the ARV drug he forgot to tell Dr. Smith about. Dr. Jones is now very worried that Fred may be at risk for the development of drug resistance due to the decreased level of the ARV medication caused by the drug-drug interaction. Having lower levels of the ARV medication in his system is almost the same as if he did not take that ARV medication.

ARV Drug Resistance: The Nemesis of Successful HIV Treatment

Remarkable advances have been made in the treatment of HIV disease over the last 30 years. The recent development of potent ARV medications that have a low pill burden and few side effects

What Nurses Know...

* *

Here are two easy ways that will help you avoid drug-drug interactions.

1. Make a list of all the medications you are on with each medication dosage. Keep that list updated, and take the list with you to every appointment you have with any healthcare provider. Be sure every healthcare provider you see (doctor, nurse practitioner, nurse, pharmacist, dentist) has an updated copy of that list and knows what medications you are taking. Be sure you also write over-the-counter medications, herbs, and supplements on the list too
2. If at all possible, get all your medications filled at the same pharmacy. That way the pharmacist can see all the medications you are taking, and if there are any potential drug-drug interactions, the pharmacist will call the healthcare providers to double-check and make sure the healthcare providers are aware and that they still want you to take the medications

has made simple medication regimens for HIV disease a reality. Despite such progress, about one-third of people living with HIV have problems taking their ARV medications as prescribed. The inability to take ARV medications as prescribed, often called non-adherence, can lead to the development of HIV drug resistance. This drug resistance makes the current regimen of ARV medications ineffective, can make other ARV medications ineffective (even if a person has never taken that ARV medication), and usually results in the need for more complex treatment regimens. The development of resistance to ARV medications is one of the biggest challenges to the successful treatment of HIV disease.

There are two ways that a person can have HIV drug resistance. The first, and least common, is to be infected with a strain of HIV from another person who has already acquired HIV drug resistance. The most common way that HIV drug resistance develops is that a person misses doses of ARV medications or starts and stops his/her ARV medications. Because HIV replicates very rapidly and has the ability to mutate (change itself), when ARV doses are missed or skipped and the level of ARV medications goes down in the blood, HIV has the opportunity to mutate and that particular ARV medication is no longer effective. When such mutations occur, the person is said to be "resistant" to a particular ARV medication or medications. HIV drug resistance typically leads to failure to suppress HIV viral load by the current ARV medication regimen.

Drug Resistance Testing

The first sign that a person either has stopped taking their ARV medications or may be missing doses of ARV medications and developing HIV drug resistance is that their viral load increases, when it was previously suppressed (undetectable). When this happens, a blood test is typically ordered to assess for HIV drug resistance. Two laboratory tests are available to detect HIV drug resistance: genotype and phenotype.

HIV genotype. A genotype test is a blood test that is used to examine the DNA of an individual's HIV strain and determine if there are mutations detected. Mutations are changes in a particular individual's strain of HIV that make that strain able to replicate in the presence of a particular ARV. Each ARV that is available to treat HIV has particular mutations, or a group of mutations, that are associated with it. If a person has HIV drug resistance, each mutation will be identified by a unique group of numbers and letters.

HIV phenotype. A phenotype test is also a blood test that is done to examine not only the presence but also the degree of HIV drug resistance. This test is typically reserved for individuals who are known to already have HIV drug resistance and may have already failed several ARV medication regimens. Phenotype tests are quite expensive and are a complicated test to run. It can often take 4 weeks to get the results.

Experienced HIV healthcare providers can interpret genotype (or phenotype) results to determine the level of drug resistance, and what combinations of ARV remain that will be effective for the individual. In general, the more HIV drug resistance mutations a person develops, the more difficult it is to construct an effective ARV medication regimen. For individuals who have chronic problems taking ARV medications faithfully and who continue to develop more and more drug resistance over time, the choices for effective regimens to treat their HIV disease become limited. For individuals with profound HIV drug resistance, treatment can require very complex ARV regimens with a number of medications and two- or three-times-a-day dosing.

The best way to prevent HIV drug resistance is to be ready to commit to taking ARV medications and to recognize adherence problems early in the course of ARV treatment. Chapter 6 is devoted to adherence. It focuses on strategies to help people who are living with HIV stick to their ARV medications faithfully. It also discusses strategies that can help overcome problems with adherence to prevent the development of HIV drug resistance and enhance health outcomes.

What Nurses Know...

HIV drug resistance can be extremely complex. The best approach is to prevent HIV drug resistance from happening by taking your ARVs faithfully every day without missing a dose. However, if you do develop resistance to ARVs, do not be surprised if the myriad of letters and numbers used to describe HIV drug resistance are a bit confusing.

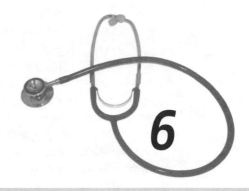

6

Staying with Your Antiretroviral Medications

I was diagnosed with tuberculosis (TB), then the doctor at the health department told me I also had HIV. I was told I needed to start on ARV medications right away because my CD4 cell count was really low. I faithfully picked up my ARV prescription every month at the pharmacy. I went to all my appointments with my nurse practitioner at the clinic. My wife went with me to all of my appointments. My TB got better but neither my wife nor the nurse practitioner could figure out why my viral load was not going down and why my CD4 cell count was getting lower. The truth was that I had not been taking any of the ARV medications. I had every bottle that I had picked up at the pharmacy hidden underneath my bathroom sink—about $10,000 worth of medications. Of course, my TB got better because the health department brought my TB medications to my house every day for 9 months and watched me take those. But as far as my ARV medications, it was up to me to take them everyday. I was in denial about having HIV and I didn't want to take medications the rest of my life. I was ashamed about what I was doing, but

I did not know what to do. I needed help. Finally one day at an appointment I confessed to both the nurse practitioner and my wife. The nurse practitioner was supportive and told my wife and me that a lot of people have trouble taking HIV medications faithfully. I found out later it's called nonadherence and that help is available if you ask for it. The nurse practitioner arranged for some sessions for me with a peer educator and she also worked with me and helped me. Today, 2 years later, I am faithfully taking my ARV medications, my viral load is undetectable, my CD4 cell count is over 500, and I am working full time. LARRY, AGE 36

Remarkable advances have been made in the treatment of HIV disease over the last three decades. Today, a person diagnosed with HIV infection can expect to live a normal life span and enjoy good health with the help of antiretroviral (ARV) medications. However, the inability to take ARV medications faithfully (called nonadherence) is a problem for many people living with HIV. Nonadherence has emerged as the major barrier to the successful treatment of HIV disease. Overcoming nonadherence is one of the most difficult challenges in the successful self-management of this disease.

Adherence: The Key to HIV Treatment Success

Untreated HIV infection causes the immune system to fail over time. Without ARV medications, HIV infection progresses to late-stage disease (called AIDS) and causes a number of health problems, such as opportunistic infections, and almost certain death. However, with ARV treatment, the complications of HIV infection are greatly reduced and the immune system can function well. In fact, ARV treatment has become so effective that universal HIV testing and immediate treatment of HIV infection with ARV medications has been proposed as a method of eliminating HIV disease worldwide.

Many research studies have shown that the key to HIV treatment success is reducing the HIV viral load to undetectable levels (suppressed HIV viral load). This goal can be reached by ensuring that a person living with HIV has full access to uninterrupted ARV medications and takes that medication every day of their lives. Missing doses of ARV medications or stopping and starting ARV medications carries a high risk for nonsuppressed HIV viral load, leading to HIV drug resistance and treatment failure. If a person develops HIV drug resistance due to nonadherence, treatment of their disease becomes more complicated. By complicated, we mean that a person will need to take more pills per day, probably several times per day. Even though there are several effective combinations of ARV medications available to treat HIV disease, the number of treatment options is limited. The newer ARV medications that are now available are a little more "forgiving" (one can occasionally miss a dose and not develop HIV drug resistance) than the medications of the 1990s. With that said, the ability to take ARV medications faithfully—every day, without missing a dose—is the key factor to ensure that a person who is living with HIV can enjoy good health and a good quality of life.

Nonadherence to HIV Treatment

While many people who receive HIV treatment are able to take their ARV medications as prescribed, about one-third (and in some communities the numbers are much higher) of people living with HIV in the United States have problems taking their HIV medicines faithfully every day. Healthcare providers cannot tell who will and who will not have problems with adherence. There are no screening tools that can predict who will be adherent or nonadherent to their ARV medications. People who are new to HIV treatment (have never taken ARV medications in the past) are thought to be the most adherent, maybe because they are more motivated or have not become "tired" of taking medications.

People who have less pills to take per day and who only need to take pills once a day tend to have an easier time "sticking to their HIV medications."

The Problem of Nonadherence

Nonadherence to HIV treatment is usually caused by several issues, not just one. The problem with nonadherence is that it leads to the development of drug resistance mutations (changes in the HIV virus itself), which make the current HIV medications ineffective. Individuals who are nonadherent to their HIV medications often have immune system decline and have symptoms of fevers, night sweats, weight loss, and diarrhea. Also, if a person is nonadherent to their HIV medications, this increases the risk that life-threatening opportunistic infections might develop (opportunistic infections are discussed in Chapter 7). Finally, untreated HIV infection (nonadherence) causes inflammation (swelling) of important body organs, such as the liver, heart, and kidneys, which can damage them. Finally, if a person is nonadherent, their HIV viral load will not be suppressed (undetectable) and this high viral load greatly increases the risk of transmitting HIV to another person through sexual contact.

The High Cost of Nonadherence

Nonadherence can make a devastating impact on an individual's health. In addition to the "cost" of nonadherence to one's health, there is also a large financial burden. As an HIV-infected person fails ARV medication regimens, not only each future medication regimen becomes more complicated (more pills, more times a day) but also the cost of the medications increases. More pills are needed, which means more copays and more possible side effects, which means more lab work, more visits to the clinic/hospital, and even more copays. While first-line ARV treatment usually involves taking one to three pills per day, ARV regimens for people with drug resistance includes taking several different pills at least twice a day. Sometimes when a person has "failed" several ARV regimens due to nonadherence and drug resistance, medications in the form of injections (giving yourself a shot) are needed. The bottom line is that as a person fails the first-line treatments and as drug resistance increases, second-, third-, and fourth-line HIV treatment becomes much more difficult and takes much more time and effort on the part of the person living with HIV disease.

What We Know about Nonadherence

There is quite a bit of information out there about nonadherence. Behavioral scientists (scientists who study human behavior) have done a lot of research and published many articles about the experience of taking ARV medications for a lifetime. It is well known that the key to success in the management of HIV disease is the ability to faithfully take ARV medications every day for a lifetime. So, for a person who has problems taking their ARV medications every day (a person who is nonadherent to their HIV treatment), becoming adherent is a life-saving behavior change. If the cycle of nonadherence can be broken, especially early on, it can mean the difference between a person living with HIV and having poor health and poor quality of life that is very costly in many ways, versus having a healthy, long and productive life. Given the importance of adherence to achieve good health, suppression of HIV viral load (undetectable viral load), and good quality of life, many studies have been conducted to better understand the behaviors of adherence and nonadherence to HIV treatment.

What Makes Taking ARV Medications Easy and What Makes It Hard?

Many issues are known to make taking ARV medications easier, or harder, for people who are living with HIV. These factors seem to be consistent for all people, regardless of things like culture, race, age, income, gender, and education level. The following are factors that have been studied by researchers and that have been found to make it easier, or harder, to take ARV medications. The factors are listed below in no particular order because everyone is different. While one of these factors may greatly impact one person, it may not impact another.

Factors that can make it harder to take ARV medications faithfully:

- Substance abuse (drugs and/or alcohol)
- Fear of disclosure of HIV status
- Denial of the HIV diagnosis
- Speaking a language different from that your healthcare provider speaks
- Stigma
- Depression
- Forgetfulness
- Suspicions about ARV treatment
- ARV medication regimens that are considered to be too complicated
- Perceived unpleasant side effects from ARV medications
- High number of pills in ARV regimen
- Sleeping through medication dosing time
- Decreased quality of life
- Work and family responsibilities
- Limited access to ARV medications

Factors that can make it easier to take ARV medications faithfully:

- Sense of self-worth
- Seeing/feeling positive effects of ARV medications
- Strong will to live
- Acceptance of the HIV diagnosis
- Understanding the need for taking ARV medications faithfully (adherence)

- Making use of reminder tools, such as pill organizers
- Having an ARV regimen that "fits" into one's daily schedule
- Once-a-day dosing schedule for ARV medications
- Being ready and motivated to take ARV medications
- Perception of a positive healthcare provider–patient relationship
- Having social support

About 6 years ago I was diagnosed with HIV. I have had the same doctor the whole time, and I think I have a good relationship with my doctor. My doctor has been worried because for the past 6 years I have only been able to get my viral load down to undetectable one time. My viral load is not too bad, but it's never undetectable and my CD4 has been slowly dropping. Finally, my doctor said he needed some help when my CD4 count dropped to 200. He asked if I was willing to talk to someone other than him about my ARV medications. He wanted me to talk to a peer educator and a nurse who specializes in adherence. They talked to me about a lot of things—not just about medicine, and I was able to tell them about things that I'd been too proud to say to my doctor. You see, one of the main reasons that my viral load was never undetectable is that some months I would miss my medicines for about a week, and then it would get to where the medicines didn't work anymore. I had drug resistance. What I had never told my doctor was that my copays for my ARVs are about $150 a month, and some months I wouldn't have the money so I didn't get my refills on time. I was too embarrassed to tell my doctor. When he would ask me if I had any problems with my medicines, I would always tell him I was taking the medicines. But talking to the peer and the nurse, that was different; they knew just the right questions to ask. And they seemed to really care about what was going on with me. As it turns out, there are two programs that can help people who have problems paying their copays. There is one program sponsored by the government and it is based on how much money you make. There are also programs sponsored by the companies that make ARV medications and many of those programs are not based on how much money you make. I qualified for help with my copays. So now I can pick up my

ARVs every month at the pharmacy without having to worry about what I will have to do without so I can make the $150 copay.   BILL, AGE 51

You Have to Be Ready

There are a lot of things in life that you have to be ready for if you are going to be successful. If you are a student and you have a test coming up and you are not ready for that test, then you probably will not do well on that test. If you are an athlete and you are not ready for the big game, you probably won't score a lot of points in that game. If you smoke and you attend a stop-smoking seminar but you really aren't ready to stop smoking, then most likely you won't be able to stop even though you went to the seminar. The same thing goes for taking ARV medications every day for the rest of your life.

Readiness for Adherence to HIV Treatment

Some people are just naturally ready to take on new challenges or endeavors—whether it is starting an exercise program, changing eating habits, or taking ARV medications every day for a lifetime. However, others need a little help getting ready to commit to big changes in their life. Although there is no single strategy to enhance adherence that can be applied to every individual, here are a few approaches, from research and clinical practice, that have worked for others. If you have tried to take ARV medications faithfully in the past but have not been as successful as you'd like, consider these things:

- Think about the issues or barriers you have experienced that have prevented you from taking your ARV medications faithfully
- Make a list of your individual barriers to adherence and then think about how you might overcome them

- Talk to people you trust, like your healthcare provider or case manager, about your barriers and ask for help in creating strategies to overcome the barriers to adherence
- Have a good relationship with your healthcare providers. It is an important part of adherence. If you do not have a good relationship with your providers, think about ways to enhance the relationship or perhaps change providers
- Have a social support that can enhance adherence, or consider joining a support group or going to a counselor if you feel you need individualized support
- People seem to do better with adherence if they have a once-a-day dosing schedule; ask your healthcare provider if this is a possibility for you
- Use a pill box. It has been found to help increase adherence
- Set a reminder device like a watch that alarms at the time you need to take your medicines, or set your cell phone to alarm, or if you are a computer user, you can set a voice reminder
- Ask for help if you have depression, problems with drinking or substance use, or feel isolated

What Nurses Know...

Experiencing problems with taking ARV therapy every day of your life is not uncommon. Living with HIV disease can be complicated and can impact not only your physical health but also your emotional health. Do not be afraid to be honest with your healthcare providers. If you are having problems taking your ARV medications as prescribed, tell your healthcare provider or your case manager. They really do want to help you.

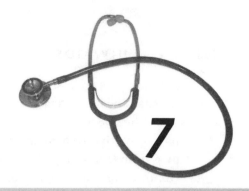

HIV-Related Infections

I had a cough that just wouldn't go away. Then I started running a temperature. I ended up going to the emergency room. I was lucky I went when I did. I ended up being admitted to the hospital. They had to do a lot of tests and then they told me I had pneumonia that only people with AIDS get. They tested me for HIV and it was positive. That was 14 years ago. I take my medicines and keep my appointments and I'm doing pretty good for an old guy. MIKE, AGE 69

The person with HIV may experience many infections during their lifetime. Some are the normal "run-of-the-mill" viruses like the common cold or a sexually transmitted infection (STI) like herpes. Other infections may be more serious because the person living with HIV may have a weakened immune system. Some of these serious infections are called *opportunistic infections* (OIs). OIs are illnesses that do not usually hurt a person with a healthy immune system. These infections do not typically occur until the immune system is very weak and the CD4 count is less than

200 cells. OIs are also called AIDS-defining conditions. A person who has an OI also has advanced HIV disease, or AIDS.

In the 1980s and 90s, OIs were very common. We did not have effective treatments for HIV disease, and many people died from OIs. Today, this type of case is rare. Now we only see OIs in people who were not diagnosed with HIV early in the course of their disease and may already have an OI when diagnosed. OIs may also occur when persons living with HIV do not get regular medical care and are not taking their HIV medications as prescribed or their medications are no longer working for them.

We are going to discuss many infections in this chapter, those that can occur at any stage of HIV and those that are considered to be OIs.

Candida is a fungal, or yeast, infection. *Candida* can cause infections throughout the body such as a vaginal "yeast" infection. People with diabetes or who have an impaired immune system, such as HIV, are more likely to be susceptible to yeast infections. It is normal to have small amounts of fungus, but when the immune system is weak, the fungus can grow, leading to slightly uncomfortable symptoms to more serious conditions. Infections from *Candida* can spread throughout your body. Following is a discussion on two types of *Candida* infections:

Thrush, or oral candidiasis, can appear at any CD4 count level. **Symptoms** include

- White patches on the gums, tongue, or inside of the cheeks
- White patches that can be scraped off with a fingernail
- Red tissue underneath the white patches that may bleed easily

If you notice these symptoms, you should contact your provider's office.

Treatment will most likely be antifungal medication. Antifungals that treat thrush come in three forms: (i) liquid medication (nystatin), (ii) lozenges that you suck on (clotrimazole), or (iii) a stronger antifungal pill (fluconazole). Normally, you only need to take these medications for a few days. If you have frequent episodes of thrush, your provider may want you to take an antifungal medicine routinely.

Esophageal candidiasis is a more serious fungal infection. It is considered an OI. *Candida* may spread to the esophagus, the tube that connects the mouth to the stomach. Persons with esophageal candidiasis will typically experience the following:

- Difficulty or pain when swallowing
- Weight loss because of difficulty eating
- Oral thrush

If you are experiencing these symptoms, you should contact your provider right away.

Your provider may want you to have an esophagogastroduodenoscopy or EGD, which is a procedure that takes a scraping from the wall of the esophagus to make certain it is *Candida.*

Treatment may include hospitalization with medications given intravenously (IV or through the vein), or treatment at home may be possible with a strong antifungal medication taken orally. The treatment method will be determined based on the seriousness of the symptoms.

Cryptococcal meningitis is a serious, potentially life-threatening OI. *Cryptococcus* is a fungus found in the soil, which is most likely inhaled through the air. *Meningitis* is an infection of the meninges, which covers the brain. It is very dangerous for people with an impaired immune system and is rarely seen in people who do not have HIV. The immune system is very impaired for this condition to occur, and the condition occurs when the CD4 count is lower than 100 cells. Symptoms include

- Fever
- Chest pain
- Fatigue

- Dry cough
- Headache
- Blurred vision
- Confusion
- Nausea and vomiting

Diagnosis of cryptococcal meningitis is made after blood, urine, sputum, and spinal fluid specimens are obtained to be analyzed in the lab. A lumbar puncture, or spinal tap, is necessary to obtain the spinal fluid.

Treatment for cryptococcal meningitis include

- Initial treatment with a strong antifungal drug (amphotericin) given through the vein
- Long-term therapy will be an oral antifungal medication (fluconazole) that needs to be taken to prevent a reoccurrence of cryptococcal disease

Cytomegalovirus (CMV) infection is a common infection that can affect anyone, often without any symptoms. In persons with advanced HIV disease, or a CD4 count less than 50 cells, it can be very serious. CMV can damage many parts of the body but most commonly causes damage to the eyes. CMV retinitis is an OI that can lead to blindness if left untreated. CMV in pregnant women can be passed to the unborn baby and may cause birth defects, or in rare cases, death. Symptoms of CMV retinitis include

- Seeing *floating spots* in front of the eye (floaters)
- Blind spots in vision
- Seeing *flashing lights*
- Loss of peripheral vision (This is the vision you have outside the central area you are looking at. Sometimes people will say they see something out of the "corner of their eye." This is peripheral vision.)
- Headaches

If you are having these symptoms, you should report them to your provider as soon as possible. Diagnosis of CMV retinitis is made by

- Having a dilated eye exam by an ophthalmologist (doctor who is an MD trained in caring for diseases of the eye) as quickly as possible. The ophthalmologist is able to identify lesions caused by the CMV
- The ophthalmologist will continue to evaluate changes to the lesions during treatment to ensure that the treatment is working the way it should

Treatment for CMV retinitis consists of two stages: the initial treatment and long-term maintenance treatment. The initial treatment is based on the severity of the disease:

- Oral medication alone (valganciclovir orally twice a day for 14 to 21 days)
- Implants containing medication (ganciclovir) are placed in the eye and the treatment may also include taking valganciclovir orally
- Intravenous (by vein) medications may be required (ganciclovir or foscarnet)

Maintenance treatment may continue life long. If the immune system improves with HIV medications and the CD4 count rises above 150 cells for more than 6 months, it is possible that maintenance therapy may be discontinued. However, your provider will want to discuss discontinuation of therapy with your ophthalmologist to ensure that your vision will not be compromised. Maintenance treatment may include

- Valganciclovir 900 mg taken orally daily
- Foscarnet IV (given through the vein) once daily

You will need to follow up routinely with an ophthalmologist to have your retinas examined for CMV disease. This is also necessary if you are taking maintenance treatment or if the maintenance treatment has been discontinued. CMV can also damage other parts of your body. If your CD4 count is less than 50 cells, you should report to your provider the following symptoms:

- Fever
- Diarrhea
- Stomach cramps
- Decreased appetite
- Weight loss
- Chest pain
- Blood in stool

Because these symptoms can also be caused by other diseases/infections, it is important to write them down and note when they started and how frequently they occur.

Hepatitis B is inflammation (swelling) of the liver caused by hepatitis B virus (HBV). The liver is a vital organ necessary for humans to survive. The function of the liver is to filter harmful substances from the blood before passing the blood on to the rest of the body. The liver has many other functions, including breaking down what you eat and turning it into energy, making proteins that are important to help the blood clot, and metabolizing drugs (the body's process of changing medications into a less toxic compound). Long-term inflammation of the liver caused by hepatitis B may result in the liver not being able to handle these functions. Although there is no cure for hepatitis B, there is a vaccine that can prevent the disease if you have not already been exposed.

Hepatitis B is a contagious disease; it spreads from person to person through contact with the blood, semen, vaginal fluids, or other body fluids. Common ways that HBV may be spread by

- Sexual contact
- Getting tattoos or piercings

- Sharing needles or drug injection equipment
- Sharing personal items, such as razors or toothbrushes
- Pregnant woman to her baby during childbirth

Hepatitis B may be an acute illness occurring within the first 6 months of exposure. The immune system is usually able to clear the virus from the body, and generally the symptoms last a short time. Hepatitis B may also become a chronic illness, which over time may cause serious liver damage. A diagnosis of hepatitis B is done by checking the following blood tests:

- Antibody to hepatitis B surface antigen: A positive result indicates you could have had a vaccination to prevent hepatitis B or you have had hepatitis B in the past
- Antibody to hepatitis B core antigen: A positive result indicates you have had a recent or past HBV infection
- Hepatitis B surface antigen: A positive result indicates you have an active hepatitis B infection
- Hepatitis B surface antigen: A positive result indicates that you have a hepatitis B infection. You could be contagious and spread hepatitis B to others through sexual contact or exposure to your blood by sharing needles. You should tell your partner(s) you have hepatitis B and discuss precautions to take with your provider

Symptoms of acute hepatitis B usually occur 2 to 3 months after exposure to HBV. Many people exposed to HBV have no symptoms. Symptoms may be mild or may be severe. Symptoms of acute HBV include

- Abdominal pain
- Dark urine
- Yellowing of skin or eyes
- Loss of appetite
- Fever
- Nausea or vomiting

- Fatigue
- Clay-colored stools

Chronic hepatitis B lasts longer than 6 months. Many times the symptoms do not become apparent for a long time, even years after the initial exposure, or the symptoms may be very mild and not thought to be of importance. People with HIV are routinely tested for hepatitis B at their first visit to their provider and usually every year following. Being routinely tested for HIV and diagnosed early may also lead to detection of other diseases, such as hepatitis B. Symptoms of chronic hepatitis B:

- Often no symptoms or mild symptoms such as fatigue or mild abdominal pain
- May develop cirrhosis or scarring of the liver. Cirrhosis symptoms include abdominal pain, nausea and vomiting, weight loss, weakness, yellowing of eyes or skin, clay-colored stools, dark urine, nosebleeds or bleeding of the gums, easy bruising, and swelling of the abdomen

Treatment for hepatitis B:

- For acute cases of hepatitis B, you may do fine and not require any treatment. You should get plenty of rest, drink plenty of fluids, and eat a nutritious diet
- For chronic hepatitis B, you will need to be regularly monitored by your provider and have blood tests done, which will help determine if liver damage has progressed. Your provider may refer you to a gastrointestinal specialist to help monitor the liver disease. Medications may be prescribed, which can help reduce the risk of liver disease or liver cancer. For very severe cases of hepatitis B, a liver transplant may be necessary
- If you do have chronic hepatitis B, you can infect other people through sexual contact or by sharing needles or drug equipment. Just as for HIV, it is necessary to use condoms, not share

needles, and tell your partner(s) that you have hepatitis B. You should also avoid sharing personal items like razors or toothbrushes, or other items that may have blood or body fluids on them, such as feminine hygiene products or sex toys. Clean up any blood or body fluid spills with bleach and water. Your sex or drug-using partners should be tested for HBV. If they have not been infected with HBV, they should be vaccinated

If you have chronic hepatitis B, here are tips for taking care of your liver. These steps may help with symptom management or prevent further damage to the liver.

- Avoid alcohol. If you have problems giving up alcohol, talk to your provider, nurse, or case manager about alcohol treatment programs
- Drink plenty of fluids and eat a healthy diet
- Avoid strenuous activities and get plenty of rest
- Talk to your provider about all the medications you are taking, including those medications that you buy over the counter, such as herbals, aspirin, or vitamins. You should also talk to your provider before you start any new medication. Liver damage may decrease its ability to metabolize medications effectively. Doses of some medications may need to be decreased and possibly discontinued
- Notify your provider if your symptoms worsen

Hepatitis C is inflammation (swelling) of the liver caused by hepatitis C virus (HCV). Hepatitis C is common in people with HIV, with some estimates of up to 30% to 40% . Just like hepatitis B, hepatitis C can be an acute or a chronic condition. Most people who are infected with HCV do develop a chronic disease. Common ways that HCV may be transmitted by:

- Unprotected sex with someone who has hepatitis C
- Sharing needles or drug injection equipment
- Receiving tattoos or piercings with contaminated equipment

- Sharing personal items that have blood or body fluids on them, such as toothbrushes, razors, or sex toys
- Pregnant women to their children
- It is possible to have contracted HCV through a blood transfusion (before 1992, as blood was not tested for hepatitis C then). Blood is now routinely tested for hepatitis C. Persons who receive renal dialysis are also at risk

There may be few or no symptoms during acute infection. If there are symptoms, there may be complaints of abdominal pain, yellowness of the skin or eyes, or fatigue. The diagnosis of HCV and decision to treat is based on results of the following lab tests:

- HCV antibody: A positive result confirms hepatitis C
- HCV RNA or viral load (which measures the amount of the virus): It is monitored for 3 months. If it is still present at 3 months, treatment may be considered. If it is still present at 6 months, the patient is determined to have chronic hepatitis C
- Hepatitis C genotype: there are six genotypes, and the type of genotype determines the treatment. Most Americans have genotype 1, which is the most difficult to treat
- Alanine aminotransferase: It helps assess liver inflammation and response to treatment
- Liver biopsy: Helps determine liver damage

Treatment of acute hepatitis C can be tricky. Coinfected patients, or patients who have both HIV and hepatitis C, may require treatment for both infections. If the CD4 count is low, the decision may be made to treat HIV first. This may boost the immune system and improve the response to hepatitis C treatment. If the CD4 count is high, then the decision may be made to give the hepatitis C treatment first, and wait to start the HIV medications. If the coinfected person is already on HIV medications, they will remain on them during the hepatitis C treatment.

Treatment for acute hepatitis C is two to three drugs given for 24 or 48 weeks. Symptoms of chronic HCV include

- Abdominal pain
- Abdominal swelling
- Fatigue
- Nausea and/or vomiting
- Dark urine
- Clay-colored stools
- Yellowing of skin or eyes
- Fever
- Itching
- Swelling of feet or ankles

A diagnosis of chronic hepatitis C is made by many of the same tests done to diagnose acute infection. Liver function tests and HCV viral loads will be done to monitor disease progression or effectiveness of treatment. The treatment of chronic hepatitis C is recommended in persons who are coinfected with HIV. Treatment of chronic hepatitis C includes the same considerations as for treatment of acute hepatitis C. Also, your provider may refer you to a gastrointestinal specialist for consultation about your hepatitis C treatment. If you have chronic hepatitis C, here are tips for taking care of your liver. These steps may help with symptom management or prevent further damage to the liver:

- Avoid alcohol. If you have problems giving up alcohol, talk to your provider, nurse, or case manager about alcohol treatment programs
- Drink plenty of fluids and eat a healthy diet
- Avoid strenuous activity and get plenty of rest
- Talk to your provider about all the medications you are taking, including those medications that you buy over the counter, such as herbals, aspirin, or vitamins. You should also talk to

your provider before you start any new medication. Liver damage may decrease its ability to metabolize medications effectively. Doses of some medications may need to be decreased and possibly discontinued

- Notify your provider if your symptoms worsen

If you have hepatitis C, you can infect people through sexual contact, by sharing needles or drug injection equipment, or by exposing them to your blood or body fluids. Just as for HIV, it is necessary to use condoms, not share needles, and tell your partners that you have hepatitis C. You should avoid sharing personal items like razors or toothbrushes, or other items that may have blood or body fluids on them, such as sex toys. Clean up any blood or body fluid spills with bleach and water. Your sex or drug-using partners should be tested for HCV.

Herpes simplex virus (HSV) is a common virus that may produce mild to severe ulcers on the mouth, genital, or rectal areas. HSV-1 is the main cause of infections that occur on the mouth and lips. These are sometimes called "fever blisters" and "cold sores." HSV-1 is contagious and can be passed to another person by kissing, sharing straws or other drinking utensils such as cups or glasses, and by oral sex. HSV-1 can also cause genital herpes. However, HSV-2 is most likely to cause genital herpes. HSV-2 is passed on through sexual contact. There is no cure for HSV infections. Once you have been infected with HSV, you will have it life long. Often, people with HSV infections experience no symptoms. The virus may go into a resting phase and be inactive, but will then become active and surface to the skin. This is when *viral shedding* may occur, which allows HSV to be passed on through sexual contact or skin-to-skin contact. Symptoms of HSV-1 may include

- Tingling or burning sensation around the mouth
- Small, painful blisters filled with fluid around the mouth or lips
- Swollen lymph nodes
- Fever
- Sore throat

Symptoms of HSV-2 may include

- Small red blistered areas or sores on or around the genitals
- Pain
- Vaginal discharge
- Fever, headache, muscle aches
- Pain when urinating

Your provider may be able to diagnose HSV infection by examining the lesions. If not, a blood test may be done to determine if you have HSV infection. This may be useful in making the diagnosis if you do not have an active outbreak. Treatment for HSV infections may be necessary to reduce the number of outbreaks and/or to relieve the symptoms. The following measures will also reduce discomfort:

- Avoid contact with the affected area before, during, and after an outbreak. You may notice a tingling sensation at the area before the outbreak occurs
- Apply ice packs or warm cloths to the area to reduce the discomfort
- If you have genital herpes, avoid wearing tight clothes or clothing that rubs against the area. Cotton underwear may be less irritating than other materials
- Antiviral medications may reduce the number of outbreaks and relieve the symptoms. These medications may be taken during an outbreak to shorten the episode or taken routinely to prevent an outbreak from occurring

Because HSV infection is contagious and can be passed on to another person even if lesions are not present, you will need to take precautions to prevent spreading HSV infection.
If you have HSV-1 infection

1. Be careful while touching your eyes or genitals
2. Do not perform oral sex

3. Avoid kissing people with sores on their lips or mouth
4. Wash your hands frequently
5. Use sunscreen to prevent further irritation from the sun
6. Reduce stress if possible. It has been linked to triggering outbreaks

If you have HSV-2 infection

1. Talk to your provider about the precautions you should take
2. Tell your sexual partner(s) that you have HSV-2
3. Avoid sexual contact when lesions are present
4. Always use latex condoms, even when you do not have an active outbreak because viral shedding may occur
5. Use a water-based lubricant to prevent friction at the area affected
6. Pregnant women with HSV infection should inform their provider, so that treatment decisions can be made to prevent transmission to the baby

Histoplasmosis is a disease caused by fungus, or yeast, which is common in the southeastern, mid-Atlantic, and central United States. *Histoplasma capsulatum* grows as a mold in the soil and becomes airborne. It can then be inhaled into the lungs. Many people are infected with histoplasmosis, but it is not a health concern unless you have a weakened immune system. It can infect your lungs, bone marrow, intestines, and other organs. For people with HIV who develop histoplasmosis, it is an AIDS-defining condition, or OI. Symptoms include

● Weight loss
● Fever
● Chills
● Headache
● Fatigue
● Cough

- Chest pain when taking in a breath
- Shortness of breath
- Skin lesions or rashes
- Mouth sores

A diagnosis of histoplasmosis is made by using urine, blood, or sputum tests, biopsies of skin, liver, or lungs may be necessary, or a lumbar puncture, or spinal tap. Treatment of histoplasmosis consists of two phases: an induction phase and a maintenance phase.

Mild to moderate histoplasmosis may be treated with oral medication (itraconazole given at a high dose) for a 3-day induction period followed by a lower dose of itraconazole taken twice a day for a total of 12 weeks of treatment. This is the maintenance phase.

A severe disease generally requires hospitalization for at least part of the treatment. During the induction phase, IV medication (amphotericin B) is given daily for at least 2 weeks, followed by maintenance therapy of itraconazole taken three times a day for 3 days, and then two times a day to complete a total of 12 weeks of treatment.

After maintenance therapy is completed, it will be necessary to continue to take a lower dose of itraconazole to prevent histoplasmosis from relapsing, or reoccurring. It is possible if your immune system improves and your blood, urine, or sputum does not have evidence of histoplasmosis that you will be able to discontinue the medication for histoplasmosis in the future.

Mycobacterium avium complex (MAC) is a group of bacteria that are related to tuberculosis (TB). However, MAC infection is not contagious like TB. This bacterial infection can make a person with advanced HIV disease very ill. It normally occurs in people with a CD4 count that is less that 50. The germs that cause MAC can be found in the environment, including food, water, and soil. Almost everyone comes into contact with MAC, but it only becomes an active disease when the immune system is not functioning as well as it should. In a person with advanced HIV disease, MAC is an OI and AIDS-defining condition. Symptoms of MAC include

- Fever—may be continuous or occur in cycles
- Night sweats
- Weakness or fatigue
- Loss of appetite
- Weight loss
- Diarrhea
- Abdominal pain
- Swollen glands (lymph nodes)

A diagnosis of MAC is reached by testing blood, urine, or bone marrow by growing a culture to check for signs of MAC. This lab procedure could take several weeks to provide a diagnosis. Other tests that could help guide your provider in making a diagnosis are blood tests that will look for other symptoms that indicate MAC, such as anemia, or not having a normal number of red blood cells.

Treatment for MAC includes using several drugs to fight the disease. Some of the medications used to treat MAC may interact with other drugs, including antiretrovirals you may be taking for HIV. Your provider will take that into consideration when deciding how to treat the MAC. Medications commonly used to treat MAC are

- Clarithromycin (Biaxin)
- Azithromycin (Zithromax)
- Ethambutol (Myambutol)
- Amikacin (Amkin)
- Rifabutin (Mycobutin)
- Moxifloxacin (Avelox)
- Rifampin (Rifadin, Rifampicin)

To prevent MAC: Your provider routinely monitors your CD4 count. If your CD4 count drops below 100 cells, your provider will discuss starting you on a medication to prevent MAC from occurring. This is called "prophylaxis," or preventing a disease from occurring. The most common medications given for MAC prophylaxis are azithromycin and clarithromycin.

Pneumocystis jiroveci pneumonia (PJP) was previously called *Pneumocystis carinii* pneumonia. PJP is caused by a fungus commonly found in the environment and does not typically cause any problems for people with a healthy immune system. However, the fungus can infect people who have a weakened immune system and cause a serious and possibly life-threatening lung infection. PJP typically occurs in people with HIV who have CD4 cell counts under 200. If your CD4 count drops lower than 200 cells, you will be prescribed an antibiotic to take routinely that will prevent PJP from occurring.

Symptoms of PJP in an HIV-positive person with a low CD4 count include dry cough, fever, fatigue/weakness, and shortness of breath; contact your provider's office immediately if you are experiencing any of these symptoms. If you are unable to contact your provider or if your symptoms worsen, you should go to an emergency department.

Diagnosis of PJP is made by chest x-ray and bronchoscopy. A bronchoscopy consists of inserting a tube through the nose or mouth to view the airways. Specimens can be taken to help identify the cause of the symptoms. Treatment for PJP most commonly includes trimethoprim–sulfamethoxazole (Bactrim). For people allergic to Bactrim or sulfa, they may be treated with pentamidine, atovaquone, or dapsone. For serious cases of PJP, steroids may also be prescribed. Persons with PJP are commonly hospitalized for a few days and then continue their treatment at home. They will usually need to take medications to treat PJP for 21 days.

As discussed earlier, you can prevent PJP from occurring by seeing your healthcare provider regularly and having your lab tests done so that your CD4 count can be monitored. If your CD4 count drops below 200 cells, your provider will want you to begin taking medicine regularly to prevent PJP. The most commonly prescribed medication for prevention of PJP is Bactrim, but if you have a sulfa allergy, you may be prescribed atovaquone, dapsone, and pyrimethamine. Pentamidine given in a breathing treatment may also be an option, but it is used much less frequently.

What Nurses Know . . .

PJP is not contagious and cannot be spread to other people. But it can be a serious, life-threatening illness in people living with HIV who have weakened immune systems and low CD4 cell counts.

To prevent PJP, you should

- Keep regular HIV healthcare provider appointments
- Have your CD4 count monitored every 3 to 4 months
- Take medications to prevent PJP as prescribed
- Report symptoms of PJP immediately—dry cough, fever, weakness/fatigue, shortness of breath

Toxoplasmosis is caused by an organism that is one of the world's most common parasites, with large numbers of people being exposed to these parasites. This parasite can be found in bird droppings, cat litter, or undercooked meat. Exposure to this parasite does not mean that you will get the disease. Toxoplasmosis can occur in persons with advanced HIV disease whose CD4 count is less than 100. A toxoplasmosis test is performed with lab work done during the initial provider visit to determine if there has been exposure to parasites. For persons in care for HIV, CD4 counts are typically monitored three to four times per year. When the CD4 count drops below 200 cells, medications, most commonly Bactrim, are given to prevent PJP from occurring. Bactrim can also prevent toxoplasmosis infection. Symptoms of toxoplasmosis include

- Headache
- Confusion
- Poor coordination (unsteady on your feet)
- Seizures
- Blurred vision
- Lung problems, such as a cough or shortness of breath

Diagnosis of toxoplasmosis may include blood tests, a magnetic resonance imaging (MRI) of the head, and a lumbar puncture or spinal tap. Treatment for toxoplasmosis includes acute (initial) therapy and maintenance therapy. The initial therapy is given for at least 6 weeks and includes taking three or more drugs, such as pyrimethamine, sulfadiazine, folinic acid, clindamycin, atovaquone, azithromycin, or Bactrim. Steroids may also be given to help decrease swelling in the brain. Seizure medications may also be necessary. Maintenance therapy includes medications that were taken during acute therapy but in a decreased dose. Maintenance therapy is usually for life but may be discontinued if the immune system improves by taking antiretrovirals and the CD4 count is over 200 for more than 6 months. MRI must also demonstrate that the toxoplasmosis lesions in the brain are no longer present. Although toxoplasmosis is not contagious, there are steps that can be taken to avoid being infected with parasites. Steps to be taken to reduce the risk of acquiring toxoplasmosis:

- Avoid eating raw or partly cooked meat. No more rare or medium steaks or hamburgers! Lamb, pork, and venison are more likely to be contaminated by parasites. Rarely, unpasteurized dairy products may be contaminated
- Be mindful not to touch your hands to your mouth while handling raw or undercooked meat, and wash your hands well when finished

- Take extra precautions when cleaning cutting boards or counters that raw or undercooked meat may have had contact with. The same is true for kitchen utensils, such as knives. Wash areas of contact and utensils with hot, soapy water; rinse well and dry
- Wash fruits and vegetables well before eating
- Ask friends or family to change the cat's litter box. If you must handle cat feces, take extra precautions by wearing gloves and a mask
- If you garden, ensure to wear gloves and wash your hands well when you are finished handling soil. You may also want to wear a mask
- While not a problem in the United States and other developed parts of the world like Canada, Europe, and Australia, toxoplasmosis may infect water supplies. If traveling to developing parts of the world, like Mexico, Africa, or Central America, drink bottled or boiled water

TB is a contagious bacterial infection that usually infects the lungs and may spread to other organs. We are only going to discuss pulmonary TB, or TB of the lungs, because it is the most common form of TB in the United States. People may be exposed to TB years earlier but not have any signs or symptoms of an active disease until their immune system becomes weakened. However, it is possible to develop active TB within weeks of being exposed. Exposure to TB most likely comes from inhaling, or breathing in, droplets from a sneeze or a cough of a person with TB. TB is a contagious infection that is a reportable condition to help protect other people from getting it. If you have TB, staff from your local health department will contact you and remain in contact with you during your treatment. Symptoms of TB include

- Cough
- Coughing up blood
- Nights sweats, may occasionally have sweats during the day
- Fever

- Fatigue
- Weight loss
- Shortness of breath
- Less frequently, chest pain

A diagnosis of pulmonary TB is made by

- Chest x-ray
- Examination of sputum specimens
- Bronchoscopy
- Blood test
- TB skin test: people living with HIV usually have this test done at their first provider visit. A TB skin test is usually done yearly thereafter to help diagnose TB early

Treatment is aimed at curing the TB infection and consists of taking several drugs for almost a year. The treatment will continue at least 6 months or longer until TB is no longer present. It is very important that you take the TB medicine as prescribed by your provider. If you do not take your TB medications as ordered, it is possible that the TB may become resistant to the medications and a more complicated, or difficult, medication regimen may be ordered. It is normal to take four different medications daily to treat TB. Commonly prescribed medications for TB are

- Isoniazid
- Rifampin
- Ethambutol
- Pyrazinamide

Less commonly prescribed medications, which may be necessary, include

- Amikacin
- Streptomycin
- Moxifloxacin

Medications used to treat TB may have side effects such as a rash or may affect the liver or vision. Before starting on TB medications, a vision test is done and instructions given that one of the medicines may cause tears or urine to be orange or brown colored. If taking that medication that changes the color of tears, contact lenses should not be worn because they will be stained with the tears. Liver tests will be done routinely during treatment to ensure that damage to the liver is detected early.

Because TB is contagious, it may be necessary to be hospitalized for 2 to 3 weeks until the medications can work to ensure that you are no longer infectious. If you live alone and remain at home, you will need to wear a mask when you go outside of your home. Family members or people who have come in contact with you will need to be tested for TB by having a TB skin test performed. If you know you have been exposed to TB, you should contact your provider immediately.

Preventing Infections from Occurring

Throughout this chapter, there has been information shared about how some of these infections can be prevented. For those infections that may have been acquired throughout your lifetime, it is important that you keep routine appointments, have labs done regularly, and report signs and symptoms of an illness to your provider, especially if your CD4 count is less than 200. Here is some general information for staying healthy while living with HIV.

Tips for staying healthy

o Keep regular appointments with your HIV healthcare provider

o Have labs done regularly, at least three to four times per year

o Report signs and symptoms of an infection or illness to your provider, especially if your CD4 count is less than 200

o Use condoms and tell your sexual partner(s) you have HIV and/or any other STI

o Practice good oral hygiene and check your mouth daily for white patches, bumps, or unusual bleeding

o Let your provider know immediately if you are aware of being exposed to TB, hepatitis, herpes, or other STI

o If your CD4 count is less than 200, take prophylaxis (medications to prevent infections) as prescribed by your provider. Let your provider know if you have side effects from these medications so that they can be changed to another medication. Do not stop taking these medications unless you discuss with your provider

o If you are taking maintenance therapy for treatment of an OI, do not stop taking those medications until you discuss with your provider. If you do stop taking those medications without consent from your provider, you risk becoming ill again from an active disease

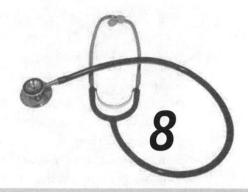

8

Mental Health and Substance Abuse

When I first found out I had HIV, I cried for days. Then I got angry that my boyfriend didn't tell me he had it. I told my case manager that sometimes I just wanted to die. She told me it was normal to go through all these changes. She hooked me up with a support group, and I met other women who already went through all this stuff. They helped me get it together, and now I help other women who go through this DOLORES, AGE 41

Mental health is how we think, feel, and act as we deal with everything that life throws at us—the good, happy times and the times that cause us stress, anger, or grief. We are frequently told how to be healthy or how to take care of our body, but being mentally healthy, especially when we are stressed, is just as important.

When you were first diagnosed with HIV, you probably experienced many emotions. You may have felt numb and unable to even focus on what you were being told about HIV. You may have felt depressed or anxious, or a combination of emotions that changed from day to day, or hour to hour. You might have felt anger at yourself for being infected with HIV or anger at the person who passed it on to you. There is no right or wrong way to feel. How one person responds is individual to them. Some people feel overwhelming sadness and cry, they even cry over things that have nothing to do with the current situation. Other people when stressed will reach for the ice cream or chocolate, hoping that "comfort" foods really do provide the comfort they are seeking. Yet others will not respond at all; it is as if nothing has happened.

Being told you have HIV is a major life event, and how you respond to it is based on your past experiences and how you have learned to cope when faced with challenges. If your usual response to stress is to use alcohol or recreational drugs, then that can of beer or bottle of gin may be what you reach for to help you through this stressful time, but it is not the healthiest way to respond and may cause more emotional pain. Alcohol and drugs may also impact your health. There are other health consequences related to how we respond to stress. Research has shown that high levels of stress may trigger an outbreak of herpes or increase the risk of reactivating the human papilloma virus in HIV-positive women. There have also been studies that indicate that some coping strategies, such as denial, may lead to a greater chance of HIV disease progression.

What Nurses Know . . .

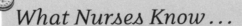

Many times, there are stages that you go through after being told you have HIV. You may go on a roller coaster ride of emotions before you are finally able to accept the fact that you have HIV and begin seeking ways to take care of yourself.

You may also have felt or will feel the same emotions when starting antiretrovirals to treat HIV, or if you are diagnosed with another chronic illness, like diabetes, or an opportunistic

- Psychologist: a person who has a doctoral degree or master's degree in psychology. Licensed psychologists are able to provide counseling, psychotherapy, and treatment for mental disorders. Most states do not allow psychologist to write prescriptions
- Licensed mental health counselor: a person who has a master's degree in psychology, counseling, or a related field and is able to evaluate and treat mental problems through counseling or psychotherapy
- Clinical social worker: a person who has a master's degree in social work and completed training that allows them to evaluate and treat mental illness. Social workers can also help advocate for patients and families
- Mental health nurse: a person who has special training in providing mental healthcare. Mental health nurses may also help advocate for patients and families and can help monitor medications

Part of the services that mental health specialists can provide you are counseling and psychotherapy. Sometimes the words counseling and psychotherapy are used interchangeably but there are differences between them. Counseling focuses on specific problems and is usually short-term therapy. Counseling helps with problem solving and learning techniques to help with coping skills. Psychotherapy focuses on a broader range of issues and seeks to help a person become aware of their subconscious patterns of thinking and learn new and healthier ways to interact with the world. It is usually a longer-term therapy.

Part of your treatment may include medications. But along with the work you are doing with a mental health professional, you can also take steps to help improve your mental health. Discuss some of these options listed below with your mental health specialist to determine which might work best for you. Here are some self-help strategies:

- Sharing or getting support from family and friends
- Make time for yourself—read a book, exercise, write, or do things that you enjoy

infection. These events may trigger a response similar to being told you were infected by HIV. The following are some of the feelings you may have or will experience. You may not feel all of them, or not feel them in the order they are listed, but they are common feelings for many people who have been told they have a chronic, and potentially serious, disease.

Denial is a common defense mechanism. It is much easier to ignore a problem or act as if nothing has happened. Being in denial for a short period of time may allow you to adjust to the news, but if it continues for an extended period of time, it prevents you from dealing with the situation and may jeopardize your health if you do not seek medical care or delay taking antiretrovirals. Signs of denial include

- Refusing to recognize a problem or situation
- Making excuses or lying about your actions, or lack of action
- Misinterpreting what others are saying or doing
- Avoidance of activities that might cause you discomfort, such as discussing HIV

Anger is a response to pain, either physical or psychological. Anger is an intense response that sends out signals to our brain that we need to fight or flee from the "thing" that is causing us pain. We usually feel other emotions before we feel anger, such as denial. Sometimes anger energizes us and readies us to fight, but anger might also become unhealthy and lead to unjustly blaming ourselves or others for the cause of our distress. Unhealthy feelings of anger may cause a desire to lash out and threaten or hurt past sexual partner(s) for giving you HIV. Unhealthy anger may also cause explosive episodes of anger over minor events. Signs of anger may include

- Fast heart rate
- Elevated blood pressure
- Tension
- Agitation

- Facial expression
- Body language
- Hostility or acts of aggression

Depression is a serious condition that can last a few days or weeks (transient) or several months or years (chronic). The person suffering depression may not be able to move forward in life, unable to make decisions, or even seek help. Signs of depression may include

- Fatigue
- Apathy or feeling indifference toward events or people that would normally cause an emotion, such as happiness, excitement, or even anger or sadness
- Difficulty focusing or concentrating
- Loss of pleasure usually experienced in daily activities
- Insomnia, or difficulty sleeping
- Changes in appetite or weight
- Feelings of low self-worthiness
- May have thoughts of suicide

Fear is a negative emotion in response to real or perceived danger, such as feeling that you will die from HIV. There might also be fear of rejection from loved ones when they find out you have HIV or AIDS. Similar to anger, it triggers the body's response to fight or flee. Signs that you are experiencing fear are similar to those of anxiety. Signs of fear include

- Increased blood pressure and heart rate
- Muscle tenseness
- Dilation of pupils
- Inability to focus

Anxiety is having feelings of panic or worry about events for which there is no need to worry or the worry is out of proportion to the cause. Anxiety may become serious enough to affect

a person's ability to do normal daily activities, such as work or attend social functions, or affect their relationships with family and friends. Anxiety can also occur when a person is depressed. Anxiety affects the way a person thinks and can also cause physical symptoms. Symptoms or signs of anxiety include

- Difficulty concentrating
- Feelings of restlessness
- Nervousness
- Excessive worry, with an unrealistic view of the cause of the worry
- Rapid heartbeat
- Sweating
- Dizziness or feeling faint
- Shortness of breath
- Headaches
- Muscle tension
- Sweaty palms
- Difficulty sleeping

Staying mentally healthy, especially during stressful times, can be very difficult. It is important that you share how you are feeling with your provider. Ongoing anxiety or depression may require medication. Sometimes your provider may recognize that you would benefit from receiving care from a specialist to help you improve your mental health. Often it takes several strategies to help you improve your mood and adjust to the stresses of life. If you do seek mental healthcare, just like your provider, a mental health specialist will become part of your healthcare team. There are different types of mental health professionals who might provide services to you based on your needs. Each can provide a different kind of service. Mental health professionals include

- Psychiatrist: a medical doctor who specializes in preventing, diagnosing, and treating mental illness and is licensed to write prescriptions

- Try meditation, Tai Chi, or yoga
- Massage
- Learn more about HIV. Having more knowledge about HIV may decrease your anxiety or depression
- If you are using alcohol or drugs, consider getting treated for your dependency
- Play with an animal. Pets give unconditional love. If you do not have a pet, or do not have friends or family nearby with pets, visit a pet store or an animal shelter
- Attend a support group

Support groups may be particularly helpful for people living with HIV. You may not be ready to talk to a group of strangers just after receiving the diagnosis of HIV, but members of support groups can provide emotional and practical support. They have been where you "are at." They have lived through many of the emotions. They can help provide information and education about HIV and support services in the area.

There are different types of support groups: a professional, such as a counselor, may facilitate some, while others may be led by a peer, or someone who also has HIV. Choose a support group that feels "right" for you. If you are uncomfortable, do not give up. Talk to your Ryan White case manager, nurse, or other healthcare provider about other support groups that may be available.

Paying for Mental Healthcare

Not all insurance companies will cover the cost of mental healthcare, or have limited treatment options. Contact your insurance company to determine the type of benefits you have, what the copays will be, and if you are restricted to specific providers or limited to a specific number of visits.

If you do not have private insurance, there may still be options for receiving mental healthcare in your area. Check if there are community-based resources, support groups, self-help groups, or public programs that may be appropriate for your needs. If you have a Ryan White case manager, they will be able to help you locate services or provide information about support groups. To find community mental health programs in your area, you can go to www.thenationalcouncil.org.

Sleep disturbances are common in people living with HIV. Actually, sleep problems are very common in the general adult population, and sometimes HIV makes sleeping problems worse. Being unable to sleep or waking several times during the night can cause fatigue or difficulty concentrating. Adults need 8 hours of sleep on an average. The best way to determine if you get enough sleep is if you wake up feeling rested and refreshed. The causes of sleep disturbances are varied and may include

- Alcohol and the use of street drugs, such as cocaine or amphetamines
- Anxiety
- Depression
- Frequent urination
- Grief
- Some medications, which may cause insomnia
- Stimulants taken before bed, such as coffee or caffeinated beverages, nicotine, alcohol, or food
- Sleeping or napping too much during the day
- Worry or stress

If you are experiencing sleep disturbances for an extended period of time, talk to your healthcare provider. There are cognitive-behavioral interventions that can be implemented to help with sleep. There are also medications that might be prescribed for a period of time to help you reset your sleeping pattern. Discuss any new prescriptions with your provider. Be certain you know what the potential side effects might be and if there are any special instructions for taking this new medication. If this medication is prescribed by a mental health professional, make certain they are aware of all medication you are taking so that no drug-drug interactions occur. You should talk to your HIV healthcare provider before starting any new medication to make certain it will not interfere with your antiretroviral.

Substance Abuse

Intravenous drug use and the sharing of intravenous needles and injection equipment is one of the causes of HIV transmission. Alcohol and other drugs also impair judgments and loosen inhibitions, leading to risky behaviors that put you in danger of acquiring sexually transmitted diseases such as HIV, herpes, and hepatitis.

People use drugs and alcohol for many reasons, but using drugs, including alcohol, impairs your thinking, which can have many serious consequences to both your health and the decisions you make. Use or abuse of alcohol and illegal drugs may begin early in childhood or as a teen. Sometimes curiosity leads to trying drugs, or because our friends are doing it. Sometimes it just sneaks up on us. We start by only drinking alcohol or doing drugs occasionally and then discover we *need* to do them more often. It does not matter how often you are doing it; if you find that your drug or alcohol use is causing problems in your life, either at work or at home, you most likely have a problem with addiction.

Alcohol is socially acceptable. We drink alcohol when we hang out with friends, to unwind at the end of the day, or to enjoy while we watch sports. Some people think having a drink will make them feel better, but the reality is that alcohol depresses the brain. When you drink to excess, your speech can become slurred and you may become less coordinated. It is humorous when you see someone else a little tipsy, sort of staggering around. But that person can easily be taken advantage of, make a decision to have sex without using a condom, and put him-/herself at risk for getting a sexually transmitted infection. Alcohol abuse is also associated with a significant percentage of motor vehicle accidents.

Alcohol can also affect your treatment for HIV or other chronic health conditions. If you have hepatitis B or C, alcohol can further damage your liver. It impacts your ability to make good decisions or to remember to do tasks, such as taking your HIV medications. Many times after drinking alcohol, you may fall asleep without even thinking about the medications you are supposed to take.

Drinking alcohol in excess can lead to alcoholism. Alcohol consumption can have a serious impact on health, causing malnutrition; liver damage; heart enlargement; and cancer of the esophagus, pancreas, and stomach. Alcohol withdrawal, either after a binge or as part of detoxification program, also poses serious health risks including anxiety, irregular heartbeat, seizures, and hallucinations. Delirium tremens can be a life-threatening condition. Most people who stop drinking alcohol will have mild to moderate symptoms that can be handled on an outpatient basis. People with a serious dependency on alcohol who stop drinking may need to be monitored by healthcare professionals in a controlled environment.

While there is no cure for alcoholism, it is a treatable condition. The first step toward beating alcoholism is to sincerely want to stop drinking. You must truly want to get help before any treatment program will work. Detoxification from alcohol may take 3 to 7 days. You should work with your provider or a detoxification treatment center to successfully detoxify without undue problems. There are outpatient and inpatient facilities that can help with alcohol and drug dependency. There are also medications that can be prescribed, which can help you remain sober. Support groups for alcoholism have proven to be very effective when combined with an established treatment program. Alcoholics Anonymous is one such program that is free and available in most communities. Talk to your provider or case manager to find a program that will work for you.

Marijuana is the most commonly used illegal drug in the United States. The smoke from marijuana is more irritating to your lungs than smoke from cigarettes and contains more cancer-causing chemicals. People often report feelings of pleasure and relaxation after smoking marijuana. However, it also impairs memory and coordination. Smoking marijuana may lead to using other drugs, such as cocaine or heroin.

Cocaine is a stimulant, which is also very addictive. Cocaine can hurt the body by causing increases in body temperature, blood pressure, and heart rate. It can cause headache, stomach pain, and nausea. People who are long-time cocaine abusers can suffer from malnutrition and paranoia. They also can experience life-threatening emergencies including heart attack or stroke.

If you use cocaine, talk to your healthcare provider or case manager about treatment options that may be available for you. You will need to work closely with a drug treatment center long term to successfully address your addiction.

Heroin is a very addictive drug that can cause serious health consequences including fatal overdose, infectious diseases such as HIV and hepatitis, abscesses, and liver or kidney disease. Women who abuse heroin during pregnancy risk delivering an infant physically dependent upon heroin and who could suffer serious medical complications.

There are treatment programs available to treat heroin addiction, including inpatient and residential treatment centers. Detoxifying along with medications and individual or group therapy sessions may be beneficial in treating heroin addiction.

Methamphetamine, or meth, is a powerful stimulant. Repeated use of methamphetamines can lead to addiction. Taking even small amounts of methamphetamines can lead to the same physical effects as cocaine. Long-term use of methamphetamines can lead to serious health consequences including malnutrition, "meth mouth" or serious dental problems, trouble sleeping, loss of memory, mood swings, and violent behavior. Methamphetamine use can alter judgment and inhibition and lead people to take risks that expose them to HIV, hepatitis, or other sexually transmitted diseases. Methamphetamine abuse can be difficult to treat. If you are using methamphetamine, please talk to your provider about treatment centers in your area.

What Nurses Know...

Remember, you do not have to overcome an addiction all alone. Your healthcare provider, case manager, and drug and alcohol counselors are there to help. Seek emotional support and comfort from family members or friends. If you have a church family, talk to your minister or other church members you are comfortable with. Recovery from an addiction can be much more successful if you are not doing it alone.

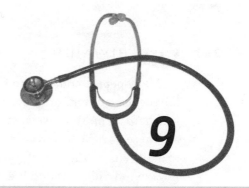

Legal Issues

When I found out I had HIV I was afraid I'd lose my job. I'm a secretary at a real estate office. My case manager told me that I didn't need to tell my boss. The only people I needed to tell were my boyfriend, my dentist, and my doctor. HELEN, AGE 30

People living with HIV have faced many social, ethical, and legal issues since the epidemic first began. Because of the widespread panic in the 1980s, many people living with HIV lost their jobs, were denied medical care and housing, and in some cases were forced to leave their communities. Fear of being infected with a contagious, and at that time, fatal disease led to discrimination against HIV-positive people, which continues to this day despite ongoing public health education about the disease. Stigma and discrimination against HIV may prevent people from having an HIV test or seeking healthcare if they are infected. There is also a concern about disclosure of their status, either intentionally or unintentionally by healthcare workers.

Many people continue to face discrimination based on color, language, religion, or gender. For many people, discrimination hits hardest on those most vulnerable, the poor.

There have been and continue to be many legal issues related to HIV. We neither are legal experts nor know about specific laws in individual states. We will try and provide you with information about some of the more common issues related to HIV, including testing, healthcare, and social services and direct you to resources that may provide you with additional information and assistance.

The Civil Rights Act of 1964 and the Americans with Disabilities Act of 1990 guarantee personal rights, among them are equal protection of the laws and protection from unlawful discrimination. These are important rights as we discuss the following legal issues.

Discrimination by Healthcare Providers

Discrimination by healthcare providers and human service providers is prohibited by laws under the Americans with Disabilities Act of 1990 and Section 504 of the Rehabilitation Act of 1973. These laws give people living with HIV the same legal protection as people with any other disability.

In 1996, the Health Insurance Portability and Accountability Act (HIPAA) was enacted. This piece of legislature ensures the privacy of patient's medical records and other health information. This includes records that may be held by a hospital, physician's office, pharmacy, nursing home, Health Maintenance Organization, or some government program. This act also ensures that patients will have access to their medical records and can control how information from their medical records is shared. If there is concern that private health information may have been released without authorization, a complaint may be filed with the Office of Civil Rights.

Making certain that these laws are enforced is the U.S. Department of Health and Human Services. Their Office of Civil

Rights is the responsible entity for enforcing these federal laws that prohibit discrimination against people living with HIV. Fact sheets from the Office of Civil Rights are provided at the end of the book. They include your rights as a person with HIV infection or AIDS, your rights under Section 504 and the Americans with Disabilities Act, your health information privacy rights, and information for filing a health information privacy complaint. For more information, visit www.hhs.gov/ocr/office.

Consent for HIV Testing

Hi Mr. Smith. Thanks for coming in for your annual exam. Today we are going to do several blood tests, including a CBC, liver tests, HIV test, and cholesterol test.

If you were recently tested for HIV, those words may be similar to how you learned you were going to have an HIV test done. Ten years ago you would (hopefully) have had a discussion with your provider about your risk factors, such as having multiple sex partners or injecting intravenous drugs, verbally agreed to an HIV test, signed a special form to have an HIV test done, and then returned 2 weeks later for the results. You might have had a lengthy conversation about what the results mean, even if they were negative, and follow-up care that should occur, including being tested again for HIV. That extensive pretest counseling, consent form, and posttest counseling were often too labor intensive for many doctor's offices to do. They did not have the time to have lengthy conversation with patients about their risk factors or they were uncomfortable discussing them. Many people with HIV were not tested early in the course of the disease.

For those reasons, in 2006, the Centers for Disease Control and Prevention (CDC) revised their guidelines regarding consent for HIV testing. The CDC no longer recommends a separate consent form be signed for HIV testing. They recommend that HIV consent be part of the general consent for medical care and that people be routinely screened for HIV. Their goal is to make HIV testing a part of routine healthcare and remove the barriers that a consent form creates. Hopefully, making HIV testing a routine procedure might reduce the stigma with which it is associated.

While patients should be told that they will be tested for HIV and given the opportunity to refuse the test (opt out), there are groups who fear that the lack of a special consent may lead to people being tested without their knowledge. There is also the possibility that stigma and discrimination will keep people from seeking care for HIV.

If you feel you were tested without your knowledge, discuss this with the provider or agency that tested you. Ask to review their policies. Your records are protected by HIPAA, and they should not release them to anyone without your consent. If you feel further action should be taken, discuss the situation with a private lawyer or contact a legal aid office near you.

Disclosure

Probably no topic is as controversial as that of disclosure. There are frequent stories in the news or newspaper about someone with HIV failing to disclose his or her status to their sexual partner. Sometimes the stories are very sensational with reports of several women or men being exposed to HIV without their knowledge. The consequences of failing to disclose your HIV status to someone who you might expose to HIV vary from state to state and can be very confusing. Many states have laws in place to prosecute individuals who knowingly expose others to HIV without their knowledge. In some states, the crime may be prosecuted as manslaughter or attempted manslaughter. These laws may also apply to spitting, scratching, or biting someone.

Important to remember is that these laws only apply to people who may come in contact with blood or body fluids. You do not have to disclose your HIV status to your relatives, employer, or people you work with.

Legal issues aside, remember how it felt to be told you had HIV. You should disclose your status to your sexual partner(s) or people you do drugs with. They need to be given the opportunity to be tested for HIV and seek medical care if necessary. If you feel uncomfortable telling them they might be at risk for having HIV, contact your local health department. They may be able to assist in contacting your partners. Also, disclose your status to your provider, dentist, or mental health worker. For you to get the best possible care, they need to know your HIV status.

Housing Discrimination

The federal Fair Housing Act ensures that people are not unfairly denied housing based on race, color, religion, national origin, sex, handicap, or familial status. In the U.S. Department of Housing and Urban Development's regulations, HIV and AIDS are considered to be an impairment and therefore protected under the Act.

If you have a Ryan White case manager, bring any forms of housing discrimination to their attention. You can also seek legal action against the landlord or file a complaint if you live in public housing. If you are worried about your safety or have been injured because of harassment, you should notify the police.

Workplace Discrimination

Although not nearly as common as it once was, there continue to be cases of discrimination in the workplace. People living with HIV are protected against discrimination in the workplace by both federal and state laws.

As mentioned earlier, people living with HIV or AIDS are protected under the Americans with Disabilities Act of 1990. HIV is qualified as a disability even if the person with HIV has no symptoms.

The Act applies to all public employers and private employers with 15 or more employees. It does not allow for discrimination in the employment practices of these employers, including hiring, application procedures, firing, training, job assignment, wages, promotions, and benefits.

If you feel you have been discriminated against in the workplace, you may file a complaint at your nearest Equal Employment Opportunity Commission Office. The complaint should be filed within 180 days of the incident.

Incarcerated Persons Living with HIV

People often comment that prisoners do not deserve any rights, and for some HIV-positive prisoners that may be the case. There have been reports of HIV-positive prisoners being segregated from the rest of the general population. Segregation may deny them opportunities that other prisoners have to shorten their prison stay through job opportunities, or access to educational and vocational programs that may help them to successfully transition back into society.

Prisoners may not be able to receive care from an HIV specialist while they are incarcerated. They may be seen by a prison physician who may not have experience or expertise in treating HIV. The prison infirmary may not stock all the available HIV medications so a person who has been receiving HIV treatment for some time may have to take HIV medications that no longer work. However, these issues are not true for all prisons.

If you feel you are being discriminated against while you are incarcerated because you have HIV, you should contact your lawyer or contact the American Civil Liberties Union. The next section provides legal resources, and fact sheets from the Office of Civil Rights are provided at the end of the book.

Legal Resources

American Civil Liberties Union: www.aclu.org
Lambda Legal Help Desk: www.lambdalegal.org
Office of Civil Rights: www.hhs.gov/ocr

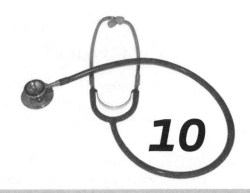

Helping a Loved One with HIV/AIDS

My oldest brother died of "pneumonia" when he was a pretty young man. Later, after I became a nurse practitioner, I figured out that all the "illnesses" he had and the reason he was so "skinny" were probably because he had HIV. I believe that what he probably died from was AIDS-related pneumocystis pneumonia.

My brother moved away from our family when he was in his early 30s and then became estranged from us. I always thought he was gay, even though he never told me. As the years have passed, my family members pretty much have all come to the conclusion that he was gay and had HIV. Many of my family members did try to reach out to him after he became estranged, but the most contact I ever got from him was a few Christmas cards with a different PO Box each year as the return address.

I think he must have been afraid that we would be ashamed of his HIV diagnosis or his sexuality or both. Or maybe he was afraid of being rejected by us—especially worried about how my "macho" Dad would deal with it. I worry that he felt very alone ... like he had a big secret that he could not share.

I wish that I would have known back then all the things that I know now about HIV disease and about how to reach out and help people with HIV disease who are having problems dealing with the diagnosis. Maybe I could have found a way to help my brother and maybe he would still be with us today. But I was just a "kid" myself back then. I didn't understand what HIV stigma was. MAITHE, COAUTHOR OF THIS BOOK

The good news is that now we know much more about HIV disease and how to help people. There are a lot of programs and many resources available that can help people learn how to accept their HIV diagnosis and that can help their families and loved ones too. Our hope is that the information in this chapter (and this book) helps the families, friends, spouses, and partners of individuals who are living with HIV. We hope it helps them to be able to reach out and connect to their loved ones who are living with HIV. We hope it can help, at least a little, to reduce the stigma that surrounds HIV. No one should have to feel like they must live in silence just because they have a disease.

It Is the HIV Stigma That Divides Us

The stigma that has surrounded HIV disease, and continues to surround it, is real and can be intense. We think stigma is the biggest reason, and maybe the only reason, that makes an individual who is diagnosed with HIV afraid to tell his/her family, friends, and loved ones about the HIV diagnosis. Stigma is also the reason that, unfortunately, families and friends sometimes reject a loved one when the HIV diagnosis is disclosed.

We do not quite understand the extreme stigma that this particular disease, HIV, carries with it. In our nursing career, we have never seen another disease that has this level of social stigma attached to it, not even other sexually transmitted infections/diseases. For example, cervical cancer caused by human papilloma virus is a sexually transmitted infection. Yet we have neither met a woman who is ashamed or feels stigmatized because she has cervical cancer nor have we ever met a family member, spouse, partner, or loved one of a woman with cervical cancer who has rejected her because of her diagnosis. The same thing goes for hepatitis B or hepatitis C, two other diseases that are acquired predominantly in the same way that a person acquires HIV.

We have spent many years asking, why this level of stigma? Over the years, older adults have told us stories about how there used to be a lot of stigma about cancer. An older lady, Gertrude, who was in her 90s told the story of her favorite aunt who got cancer when Gertrude was just 12. Gertrude was never again allowed to see her aunt and then her aunt passed away. Gertrude has regretted being isolated from her aunt all her life. Gertrude said that cancer stigma went away when people started learning more about cancer, learning more about how people got cancer, learning that you cannot "catch" cancer just by talking or hugging someone, learning more about the treatment for cancer, and figuring out that cancer was not necessarily a death sentence. So that is why we have stopped asking "why?" and instead made a commitment to try and help people learn about HIV, learn about how people "get" HIV, help them understand that you cannot get HIV from talking to people with HIV, from hugging people with HIV, from being friends with people with HIV, and that there is great treatment available for HIV disease so that people who do have HIV can live long, healthy, and productive lives. That is one of the reasons when we were asked to write this book, we said YES! This book is another opportunity to break down the stigma that surrounds HIV. So after you have finished reading this book, we hope you will pass it on to another person and ask them to read it too, and then keep passing it on.

Silence Is Not Golden

The best way to break down HIV stigma is to talk about it. If you or someone in your circle of family or friends has a "phobia" about HIV, then you have to find a way to talk about HIV and to get past issues surrounding HIV. You should do this for the benefit of your loved one who is living with HIV. You should do this for yourself. And you should do this for the benefit of the millions of people in this world who are living with HIV and who are suffering because they feel stigmatized by this disease—a disease, by the way, that is treatable and can be successfully managed for a lifetime. No one should have to live with a lifetime of stigma. The best way to get over a "phobia" is to have an honest conversation about it. Start by having a conversation with yourself.

We have had a number of people tell us over the years that "those people" (who have HIV) are drug addicts and prostitutes. Unfortunately, we still hear these types of statements today. Despite all the money, time, blood, sweat, and tears that have been devoted to HIV education, many people still think that a person has to engage in very "risky" behaviors to acquire HIV. The truth is, most people "get" HIV by having sex with someone they really care about: usually their partner, boyfriend, girlfriend, husband, or wife. Most people do not know that, on a global level, one of the biggest risk factors for women acquiring HIV is marriage.

So, we think the first step to getting past any issues that people may have about HIV disease is to think about the fact that most people "get" HIV by having sex with someone they care about. Second, remember that people are sexual beings, and sex is a normal and needed human behavior. Third, remember that most people are having sex or have had sex sometime in their life. Let us be really honest with each other: if our parents had never had sex, I would not be writing this book, and you would never have the chance to read it.

Can we be even more honest with ourselves? How many couples do you know who were virgins when they entered into their sexual relationship and that remain in that same monogamous sexual relationship? Have you only had sex with one person in your whole life? And if yes, are you sure that person was a virgin when you entered into the relationship? The truth is that most people have had sex with more than one partner, most people have had unprotected sex at some point in their lives, and many of us were just "lucky" if we never acquired a sexually transmitted infection or had an unintended pregnancy or got HIV.

Now let us go even one step further. What about all the people in this world who have acquired HIV in utero—those are the individuals who were born to HIV-infected mothers and acquired HIV simply by being born. Why should innocent children who have not engaged in any type of "high-risk" behavior be stigmatized for having a disease that he/she could never have prevented? So, we think it is worth repeating: the first step to ending HIV stigma and getting over any "phobia" is to have an honest conversation. Start by having it with yourself and then start having the conversation with your family, friends, and anyone who will listen. If enough of us have this conversation, we can put an end to HIV stigma.

Relationships Change When a Loved One Has HIV

Most of our patients tell me—the ones who have disclosed their diagnosis to their loved ones—that they just want their loved ones to treat them as they are "normal." To do "normal" things with them like watch TV, play games, or go for a walk and to forget about the HIV. But what usually happens is that after a loved one, family member, or a friend finds out that a person they care about has HIV, they treat them "different" than before the diagnosis. Reactions and behaviors of partners, spouses, families, and friends can range from one extreme to the other: from shutting the person who has HIV out of their life to smothering the person with attention and everything in between. But inevitably there is a change in people's behaviors, and the dynamics of relationships change after the HIV diagnosis is disclosed.

The first reaction, usually, is that partners/spouses/family/friends fear that their loved one will die. Actually, most of the time, the person who is diagnosed with HIV feels that way at first too, especially right after the diagnosis is made. Then, the stigma usually sneaks in and brings with it lots of questions. Emotions are flying about "how" the person "got" HIV. As a nurse practitioner who has devoted my practice to the care of people who are living with HIV, I never ask my patients how they "got" HIV. From my perspective, it does not matter. My job is to take care of the person, help them learn how to enhance their health, and make sure they know how to protect their own sexual health and to protect the sexual health of others. However, most of the time, patients spend a lot of time telling me how they did, or did not, get HIV and asking me if I can figure out exactly how they got HIV or if I have a test to figure out who they got HIV from. The answer is that there is no test that can tell us how a person acquired HIV infection. There is not even a test that can tell us exactly how long a person has been infected with HIV. The diagnostic tests we have only tell us that a person is infected with HIV —not how, when, or where the infection was acquired.

Getting Started

It is easy for us to sit here, after many years of experience, and write about how you should be going out and talking about HIV and sex. Actually, it may be pretty easy to talk to yourself about sex, but after that it definitely gets more difficult. Honestly, these are really tough topics to talk about with other people: especially if those other people are your family members and if you are from a family like mine where no one has ever talked much about sex or any other "deep" topic.

Learn All You Can

One of the best ways to start the conversation about HIV is by learning all you can about HIV. Obviously you are reading this book, so your quest for knowledge has already begun. Be sure you learn from sources that are reliable and provide up-to-date and accurate information. This book contains a resource list of trusted Web sites. Many libraries have health librarians who can also point you to trusted information sources. If you live in a city with a public university, you can go to that university's health sciences library and ask the librarian to help you find information. Below is a list of people and places where you might go for help and also to learn more about HIV.

Your Loved One's Healthcare Provider

Ask your loved one if you can go with them when they see their HIV healthcare provider. If your loved one does not feel comfortable having you in the room with them while he/she is seen by their provider, maybe you can start by just going to the appointment and sitting in the lobby. Depending on the place where your loved one receives care, you may learn a lot just by sitting in the waiting room. Many clinics that provide HIV care have brochures, magazines, and other materials right in the lobby or on bulletin boards. If you do go into the room while your loved one sees their healthcare provider, ask the healthcare provider if there is anything that he/she thinks you could do to help your loved one. Usually when my patient's loved ones ask me that question, I reply by saying that just by coming to the appointment they have already helped. Then I load them up with brochures, pamphlets, magazines, and handouts about HIV and about any upcoming community programs. I always tell loved ones that they are welcome to come to any and all appointments because HIV is a disease that requires not just medicine, but a lot of social support to ensure good health outcomes.

Your Loved One's Case Manager

Ask your loved one if he/she has a Ryan White case manager. If not, encourage them to explore getting into Ryan White case management. More detailed information about Ryan White case management is available in Chapter 2. Ryan White case managers are a wealth of information and their services are government sponsored, which means they are free for your loved one and for you. Ask to meet with your loved one and his/her case manager. Just like meeting your loved one's healthcare provider, this will be another opportunity to provide support, to learn more about your loved one's disease process, and to ask how you can help.

AIDS Service Organizations

Find out if there is an AIDS service organization (ASO) in your community. If there is, check it out. ASOs are typically grass-roots, not-for-profit organizations that were started in response to the AIDS epidemic. Many began as a group of volunteers who gathered together in a church basement or someone's home. Services provided by these organizations vary widely and can include prevention, advocacy, outreach, HIV treatment, respite care, and comprehensive care. Most are community-based organizations that are governed by a board of directors from the community. ASOs often provide programs and services with a mix of public and private funding. To find ASOs in your community, ask HIV healthcare providers or case managers, or you can even do an Internet search.

Support Groups

What we have learned from many years as nurses taking care of people who are living with HIV disease is that one of the best and most meaningful types of social support comes from other people who are also living with HIV disease. Being with other people who are familiar with HIV disease because they have lived it is the absolute best. This type of interaction lets a person know that he/she is not alone and makes for a conversation between people who are in the same life situation. A diagnosis of HIV bonds people. We have had patients who are doing very poorly with their HIV self-care management do a 180-degree turnaround when they make a bond with another person who is living with the disease, and this bond does not have to necessarily form between two people who have anything else in common. One of our favorite stories is about a 20-something gay Black male living with HIV who got to know a 40-something Latina mother of two living with HIV at an educational program we had for patients of our clinic. The only thing the two of them really had in common was HIV, but that was enough. They formed a bond that became a support system for themselves, and later for others.

Encourage your loved one who is living with HIV to consider attending an HIV support group or getting involved in a structured support program. Ask your loved one's healthcare provider or case manger for a referral to a support group or look into structured education and support programs funded by federal, state, or local government. One such program is L.I.F.E. (Learning Immune Function Enhancement), a program that has been around since 1974. Many of our patients have completed the L.I.F.E. program and have said it was extremely helpful for them. Many communities offer the L.I.F.E. program free of charge. For more information about L.I.F.E., go to www.shanti.org or ask your Ryan White case manager.

We have discussed support groups earlier in this book, but it cannot be said enough. Support groups and structured support programs are an excellent way to help individuals who are living with HIV cope with the stressors of having a chronic disease. In particular, because HIV is a disease that has a certain amount of social stigma attached to it, having social support can help your loved one (and you) to accept the diagnosis, take care of his/her health, and have a higher quality of life.

Educational Programs and Conferences

Consider attending an HIV educational program or conference with your loved one, or alone, to learn more about the disease. Local ASOs and HIV healthcare clinics often host community programs about many aspects of HIV. Ask your loved one's case manager or healthcare provider about local programs that are offered in your community.

National and regional conferences are another valuable source of information. Such conferences may offer reduced registration fees for HIV-affected individuals who attend. Look for annual conferences offered by reputable organizations such as

- AIDS Education and Training Centers at http://www.aids-ed.org
- Infectious Disease Society of America at http://www.idsociety.org
- Association of Nurses in AIDS Care at http://www.nurses-inaidscare.org
- International Association of Physicians in AIDS Care at http://www.iapac.org
- International AIDS Conference (held every 2 years) at http://www.aids2012.org

Faith-Based Organizations

Your local churches and faith-based organizations are another place to look for help. Programs, such as the National Week of Prayer for the Healing of AIDS (formerly the Black Church Week of Prayer for the Health of AIDS), that focus on raising awareness and helping individuals in their community who are living with HIV are very active in many churches. To learn more about this endeavor, or to find a church that participates in the National Week of Prayer, go to http://www.nationalweekofprayerforthe-healingofaids.org.

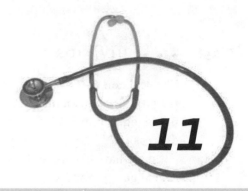

Your Love Life

Ever since I found out I was HIV positive, I haven't been with any-
one. I don't want to be with anyone because I don't want to give
this to anyone. I moved in with my Mom a couple of years ago and
help take care of her in her old age. I just go to work and stay to
myself ... I'm very lonely.   BERT, AGE 50

For people living with HIV, having this diagnosis can significantly impact the quality of their love life. Usually right after
the diagnosis, there is a period of emotional turmoil. There
are a lot of questions. People start thinking about how their
HIV infection was acquired. They may be angry at the person
who transmitted the HIV. They may start asking "why me?"
Eventually, the issue of sex and having intimate relationships
presents itself.

Some people choose not to have any more intimate relationships once they have been diagnosed with HIV. While this usually
sounds like the easiest and most practical solution to solving the
issues and problems about sex and intimacy, it usually does not.

The decision to shut the door on the thought of ever even having the possibility of an intimate relationship, and become a nonsexual being, often results in loneliness, isolation, and sometimes depression.

As we have discussed in other parts of this book, humans are sexual beings and having intimate sexual relationships is a normal part of life. It is important to know that you can have a love life as a person who is living with HIV. This chapter discusses how to have an active love life while protecting your sexual health and your partner's sexual health, too. We do not believe that HIV is a reason for you to cut off the notion of ever having an intimate relationship. We are all human and sexual beings, and we need and deserve intimacy. However, it is important to find the "right person" and to protect your sexual health, the other person's sexual health, and your emotional health as well. So, before you decide to pursue an intimate relationship as a person living with HIV, it is important to have all the information you need about sexually transmitted infections (STIs) and the skills and tools to protect your sexual health.

In addition, for many reasons, it is important to tell your potential sexual partner(s) that you have HIV infection, before you become intimate with that person. Not telling a sexual partner your HIV status is a crime, and in most states having unprotected sex and transmitting HIV to another person is a felony.

How to Protect Your Sexual Health

For the sexual transmission of HIV and most STIs to occur, there must be an exchange of semen or vaginal fluids. HIV cannot be transmitted by hugging, kissing, touching, or any other type of casual contact.

ABSTINENCE
The safest way to protect your sexual health is to not have intercourse or oral sex. It is possible to have an intimate relationship and still abstain, in other words not to exchange semen and

vaginal fluids. We have had many couples tell us that they are perfectly happy with abstinence and that they have found other creative fun ways to have a love life, without exchanging semen or vaginal fluids with their sexual partner. Their successful strategies have included such things as the use of sex toys, mutual masturbation, or just simply cuddling.

BARRIER PROTECTION

For couples that do decide to have intercourse and/or oral sex, barrier protection is the best way to prevent the exchange of body fluids and protect your sexual health. Latex condoms that cover the penis (male condoms) offer significant protection (not 100%) to prevent the exchange of semen during sexual activity. Male condoms come in a variety of colors and also come in more than one size. Female condoms are also available and this type of condom covers the vagina. The penis is inserted into the female condom during intercourse. Male and female condoms should not be used at the same time because they can curl up on each other and become ineffective. The same goes for using more than one condom at a time. Whether using a male or a female condom, it is important to use plenty of water-soluble lubricant with the condom. There are quite a few brands of excellent lubricant available at most stores that sell condoms, such as Wet and RAIN. For vaginal oral sex, a dental dam can be used to prevent vaginal fluids from entering the mouth. Dental dams can be purchased (although they can be hard to find at stores) or you can make a dental dam from a nonlubricated condom. To make a dental dam from a condom, cut off the top rounded part and then cut it down the long end so that it then becomes a square barrier that can be placed over the vagina. There is a video available on YouTube that demonstrates how to make a dental dam from a condom.

Sexually Transmitted Infections

Bacterial vaginosis (BV) is a condition that occurs in women. There is a disruption in the normal balance of "good" bacteria

What Nurses Know...

Even if both people in a sexual relationship are HIV infected, they should still avoid exchanging semen and/or vaginal fluids. There are two reasons. The first is to prevent the transmission of STIs, other than HIV, from one person to the other. The second is to prevent reinfection of HIV with a strain of HIV that might be drug resistant or more virulent than the other person's HIV strain.

in the vagina and it is replaced by an overgrowth of "bad" bacteria. The cause of BV is not completely understood, but is seems to occur more often in women who have a new sexual partner, have multiple sexual partners, or who douche. Symptoms of BV include a vaginal discharge that smells "fishy," burning during urination, and/or itching. BV is treatable with antibiotics. BV can recur after treatment. If you think you have symptoms of BV, you should see a healthcare provider.

Chlamydia is the most commonly reported STI in the United States. It is caused by the bacterium, *Chlamydia trachomatis.* For women, symptoms of chlamydia are usually mild or absent. However, serious complications that cause irreversible damage, including infertility, can occur if left untreated. For this reason, many women's healthcare providers routinely screen women for chlamydia during cervical cancer screening (Pap testing). Chlamydia also occurs in men and can cause discharge from the penis. Among men, the discharge is what usually leads to seeing a healthcare provider and making the diagnosis. Chlamydia can be easily treated, and cured, with antibiotics. If you think you have symptoms of chlamydia, or that you have been exposed to chlamydia, you should see a healthcare provider.

Genital herpes is an STI caused by herpes simplex virus (HSV) type 1 or type 2 that occurs in both men and women. Most cases of genital herpes are caused by HSV-2. Many people have HSV infection but have no or minimal symptoms. When symptoms do occur, they present as a "break out" of tender, painful blisters in the genital area, on the penis or the rectum. Genital herpes is the most common STI. It occurs in one out of six people in the United States and is more common in women. There is no cure for genital herpes, but taking antiviral medications can help prevent and reduce the number of breakouts.

Genital herpes can be transmitted even when there are no symptoms present. Condoms are not highly effective in the prevention of transmission of genital herpes.

If a woman contracts genital herpes or has a breakout during pregnancy, it can be life-threatening for the baby if the baby becomes infected. For this reason, women with genital herpes usually have a cesarean section.

Gonorrhea is an STI caused by *Neisseria gonorrhoeae* and occurs in both men and women. In women, gonorrhea can infect the cervix (opening to the womb), uterus (womb), and fallopian tubes (egg canals). In men, it can infect the urethra (urine canal). Gonorrhea can also infect the mouth, throat, eyes, and anus.

In men, symptoms usually appear within 1 to 14 days after infection; however, some men have no symptoms at all. Common symptoms of gonorrhea are burning sensation during urination, a discharge from the penis, and sometimes painful, swollen testicles. In women, the symptoms of gonorrhea are usually mild, but most women who are infected have no symptoms. For this reason, many women's healthcare providers routinely screen women for gonorrhea during well-woman examinations/cervical cancer screening (Pap testing). Symptoms in women can include a painful or burning sensation when urinating, increased vaginal discharge, or vaginal bleeding between periods. Symptoms of rectal infection in both men and women may include discharge, anal itching, soreness, bleeding, or painful bowel movements.

However, rectal gonorrhea infection may cause no symptoms at all. Infections in the throat may cause a sore throat, but usually there are no symptoms. Treatment is available for gonorrhea, and it can usually be cured with antibiotics.

Human papillomavirus (HPV) is a very common STI. There are more than 40 HPV types that can infect the genital areas of men and women; the mouth and throat can also be infected. HPV is most often transmitted through vaginal or anal intercourse. In most cases, HPV infection does not cause any symptoms because the immune system clears the infection. However, certain types of HPV can cause warts around the genital area, rectal area, or mouth. Of greatest importance is the fact that certain types of HPV are the causes of cervical or anal cancer. While there is no cure for HPV, there is a vaccine available to prevent infection with the HPV types that most often cause cancer or genital warts. The HPV vaccine is recommended for individuals aged between 11 and 26. The HPV vaccine has not yet been approved for individuals with HIV infection.

What Nurses Know...

Genital and anal HPV infection is very common, and certain types of HPV can cause genital and anal cancer. It is very important for all people who have been sexually active to have routine annual screenings for cervical cancer and anal cancer. It is especially important for people living with HIV disease to have annual cervical cancer and anal cancer screenings because there is a higher rate of cervical and anal cancer from HPV among people with HIV disease.

Syphilis is a sexually transmitted disease (STD) caused by the bacterium *Treponema pallidum* that affects both men and women. The symptoms of syphilis can sometimes be difficult to figure out because many of the symptoms can be similar to other health conditions or can be minor and overlooked. Syphilis occurs in three stages: primary, secondary, and late stages. In the primary stage (first 10 to 90 days after infection), there is typically a sore that occurs in the genital area, but the sore can also occur in other places on the body and there can be more than one. If syphilis is not diagnosed in the primary stage, then as the sore(s) is healing or several weeks after the symptoms of sore(s) go away, then a rash will occur. In this second stage, the rash can be serious and be accompanied with fever or swollen lymph nodes, or the rash can be minor and a person may not even notice it. Then if there is no diagnosis or treatment, 10 to 20 years later, late-stage syphilis can occur. In the late stages, syphilis can do damage to vital organs and even lead to death. The good news is that syphilis is easy to cure with antibiotics if diagnosed in the early stages and can still be treated later in the disease process before complications of late-stage syphilis set in.

Trichomoniasis is a common STD that affects both women and men; however, symptoms are much more common in women. Trichomoniasis is caused by the protozoan parasite, *Trichomonas vaginalis,* and the vagina is the most common site of infection in women. For men, the urethra (urine canal) is the most common site of infection. Trichomoniasis is sexually transmitted through penis-to-vagina intercourse or vulva-to-vulva (the genital area outside the vagina) contact with an infected partner. Women can acquire the disease from infected men or women. Men usually contract trichomoniasis only from infected women. Trichomoniasis is usually not a disease of men who have sex with men, unless they are bisexual. Most men with trichomoniasis do not have signs or symptoms. Women can have symptoms of infection that include a frothy, yellow-green vaginal discharge with a strong odor. It can also cause discomfort during intercourse and urination, and irritation and itching of the female genital area. Trichomoniasis is diagnosed with a lab test, and the infection can be cured with antibiotics.

What Nurses Know...

If you think you have symptoms of any STI, or you think that you have been exposed to one, you should see your health-care provider as soon as possible. You can also get screening, examination, diagnosis, and treatment for STIs, usually for free, at your local health department. Putting off screening and treatment of STIs can lead to irreversible problems, such as infertility, and also increases the risk of transmitting the STI to another person.

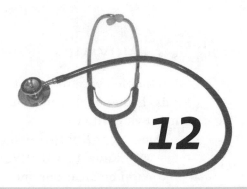

12

Men's Health

Before I got diagnosed with HIV, I never went to the doctor. Well, I mean I only went if I was really sick or had a cut or a broken bone or something like that.   MARIO, AGE 43

Over the years, when we have volunteered at many health fairs that offer health screenings and information about wellness and prevention, it seemed there were always more women than men. We have staffed many health and wellness fairs at shopping malls and churches and given information to check blood pressure, blood sugar, and cholesterol of many women. Perhaps it is different in your community, but in ours, unless mama or *abuela* (grandma) brought the men in, they just did not come.

This chapter is devoted to men's health and is full of information about health screenings and prevention tips for men. We hope the men, and women, reading this book will share this information with the men they love. Most of the information in this chapter applies to all men, with caveats that are specific to men living with HIV.

Most of the people living with HIV in North America are men. We know that if HIV-infected men have access to anti-retroviral medications and are faithful to their HIV treatment every day of their lives, they can expect to live a long life into their 60s and 70s. Today, the majority of men who are living with HIV do not die from complications of HIV alone. So, it is very important for men who are living with HIV to pay attention to other aspects of their health, not just their HIV disease. The top causes of death for men of all races in the United States, regardless of HIV status, are heart disease and cancer. Together, heart disease and cancer account for over 50% of the deaths among men.

Many of the things that threaten men's health are preventable. The Centers for Disease Control has complied data about the seven top causes for poor health among all men. This chapter focuses on those top causes and provides strategies and "tips" to prevent them, plus information about many other important men's health issues. You will soon see that many of these tips are the same for a lot of men's health risks that are discussed in this chapter. As you are reading, remember that the key to good health is to stay on top of your health— it is the best way to keep it!

The Top Seven Threats to Men's Health

HEART DISEASE

Heart disease is a leading killer of men. Here are some things you can do to take charge of your health.

Do not smoke. If you smoke or use other tobacco products (chew, cigars), ask for help so you can quit. Ask your healthcare provider, your case manager at your local hospital, or community health center. There are many programs, and some are free, that can help you quit smoking. Also remember to avoid secondhand smoke.

Eat healthy foods. Eat plenty of vegetables and fruits (fresh or frozen) together with whole grains, high-fiber foods, and lean sources of protein, such as fish. Cut down on foods that are high in saturated fat and sodium (avoid greasy, fried, and salty foods).

Know your cholesterol, blood pressure, and blood sugar. If you have high cholesterol, high blood pressure, or diabetes, keep them under control through a healthy lifestyle (diet and exercise) and taking medications if needed.

Be active every day. Get up off the sofa. Walk more, join a sports team or other activities you like, such as basketball, football, or tennis.

Maintain a healthy weight. Lose those extra pounds; they increase the risk of heart disease.

Limit alcohol. If you choose to drink alcohol, do so only in moderation. Too much alcohol can raise your blood pressure.

Manage stress. If you constantly worry, are "on edge," or can not sleep due to stress, ask for help and find ways to reduce your stress. Ask your healthcare provider, case manager, or pastor if you belong to a church. There are many community programs to help people manage their stress in healthy ways.

CANCER

There are several cancers that affect men: lung cancer, prostate cancer, colorectal cancer, and skin cancer. Anal cancer is of particular risk for men living with HIV who have sex with men. Here are some general tips for men about how to reduce the risk for cancer.

Do not smoke. Any type of tobacco use puts you at risk for cancer. If you smoke or chew, get help and quit. Also remember to avoid secondhand smoke because it is just as much of a risk.

Maintain a healthy weight. Lose those extra pounds, and keep them off—it may lower the risk for several types of cancer.

Be active. Physical activity will help keep you at a healthy weight, and just the physical activity on its own may lower the risk of certain types of cancer.

Keep those fruits and veggies coming. While eating healthy is not a guarantee as far as cancer prevention, it may help reduce your risk.

Protect your skin from the sun. When you are outside, cover up and use plenty of sunscreen.

Limit alcohol. If you drink, do it in moderation. For several types of cancer—colon, lung, kidney, and liver—the risk of cancer increases with the amount of alcohol you drink and the length of time you have been drinking regularly.

Get serious about early screenings. Get cancer screenings early and before symptoms appear. Early detection saves lives and it is the key to preventing and curing cancers. There is a section later in this chapter about cancer screenings specific to men and men with HIV disease.

ACCIDENTS

Car accidents are a leading cause of death among men. Use common sense and stay safe on the road. Wear your seat belt. Follow the speed limit. Do not drive under the influence of alcohol or any other substances or when feeling sleepy. And please do not text or talk on your cell phone while driving.

CHRONIC LUNG DISEASES

Lung problems like bronchitis and emphysema are a major health concern for men. Here are some tips to protect your lungs.

Do not smoke. If you do smoke, ask for help so you can you quit. Also avoid exposure to secondhand smoke.

Stay away from pollution. Stay away from exposure to chemicals and outdoor air pollution.

Prevent lung infections. Wash your hands often. Get vaccinated for flu (every year) and pneumonia (given twice, once at baseline and the other 5 years later).

STROKE

There are some risk factors for stroke that cannot be controlled. These include your family history, age, and race, but there are quite a few others that you can control.

Cholesterol, blood pressure, and blood sugar. Be sure you know what your cholesterol, blood pressure, and blood sugar levels are. If you have high cholesterol (hyperlipidemia), high blood pressure (hypertension), or high blood sugar (diabetes), get them treated and keep them under control.

Do not smoke. If you do smoke, ask for help so you can quit.

Eat a healthy diet. Limit foods high in saturated fat and cholesterol (like greasy, fatty, fried foods).

Keep moving. Include physical activity in your daily routine. If you are overweight, start working on losing those extra pounds.

Limit alcohol. If you choose to drink alcohol, drink in moderation.

TYPE 2 DIABETES

There are two types of diabetes: type 1 and type 2 diabetes. Type 1 is the diabetes of childhood and usually occurs in young children. Type 2 diabetes is the most common type of diabetes and usually starts in adulthood, but it can start in children later in their preteen and teen years.

Type 2 diabetes is a health problem that affects the way your body processes and uses blood sugar (glucose). High levels of blood sugar (poorly controlled diabetes) can lead to heart disease, eye problems (including blindness), nerve damage (diabetic neuropathy), and kidney problems (including kidney failure).

To prevent type 2 diabetes, get serious about your eating and lifestyle habits. Eat healthy and exercise and lose those extra pounds.

SUICIDE

Suicide is another leading risk to men's health. Depression is an important risk factor for suicide among men. If you have signs and symptoms of depression—feelings of sadness or unhappiness, loss of interest in normal activities, trouble sleeping, crying frequently—talk to your healthcare provider. Help and treatment are available. If you are thinking about suicide, call 911 or go to the nearest emergency room.

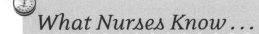

What Nurses Know . . .

It is hard to change lifestyle habits, but do not feel intimidated. Instead, do whatever you can to lead a healthy lifestyle. Start with small steps; instead of drinking soda every day with lunch, start drinking water. Instead of taking the closest parking spot to the front door, choose a spot that is a little farther away and walk a few extra steps—those types of small steps will lead to bigger steps. Simple preventive measures can go a long way toward reducing your health risks.

Men-Specific Health Issues

PROSTATE CANCER

Most prostate cancer is discovered through routine screening. There is some controversy among health experts about when to start screening or if prostate cancer screening should even be done. Most healthcare providers recommend men start prostate cancer screening in their 50s, or sooner for men who have a family history or other risk factors for prostate cancer. It is important to know the risk factors for prostate cancer and the reasons that you should see a healthcare provider about your prostate health:

- Trouble urinating
- Decreased force in the stream of urine
- Blood in the urine

- Blood in the semen
- Leg swelling
- Pain/discomfort in the pelvic area
- Bone pain

ANAL CANCER

Screening for anal cancer is pretty new. Anal cancer is much more common in individuals who are living with HIV and it is of particularly high risk for men who have sex with men who are HIV infected. Anal cancer, like cervical cancer in women, is caused by human papillomavirus. Anal Pap testing and high-resolution anoscopy (HRA) are the two screening tests available for anal cancer. Men living with HIV should be screened for anal cancer once a year.

Anal Pap Test

A Pap smear, also called a Pap test, is a screening procedure to test for atypical (odd) or cancer cells of the anus. You may have heard of a Pap test from your women family members or friends. The Pap test has been around for many years as a life-saving screening test for cervical cancer. The anal cancer screening Pap test is almost identical to the Pap smear test that involves collecting cells from the cervix of women. The anal Pap test involves collecting cells from the anus using a soft swab (it looks like a long Q-tip).

Early detection of anal cancer or atypical cells that could lead to anal cancer gives you a greater chance to prevent, or cure, anal cancer. A Pap test can also detect changes in your cells that suggest cancer may develop in the anus in the future. Detecting these cells early with a Pap test or HRA is the first step in stopping the development of anal cancer.

High-Resolution Anoscopy

All abnormal anal Pap tests must be followed up with an HRA procedure. HRA is emerging as the "gold standard" for anal cancer screening. Many experts feel that anal Pap testing will be eliminated and HRA will become the screening mechanism of choice for anal cancer. HRA is a procedure that examines the anus using an instrument called an anoscope. During anoscopy, a sample of tissue (biopsy) is usually collected and sent for further laboratory testing. If you have an abnormal anal Pap and are asked to have an anoscopy, this does not necessarily mean you have cancer. But it is important to follow all abnormal anal Pap tests with anoscopy because detecting abnormal cells, or cancer cells, early on results in the best chance to stop cancer from developing or to cure the cancer.

Many men experience anxiety before their anal Pap or anoscopy exams. Knowing what to expect during your anal cancer screening tests may help you feel more comfortable. Before you have anal cancer screening, ask your healthcare provider to explain the procedure to you step by step. Anal Pap testing and HRA are procedures that are done in the office (outpatient) setting and do not require anesthesia. You can drive yourself to/from the appointment.

OTHER CANCER SCREENINGS

There are several tests available to screen for colon cancer. The most common screening test is called colonoscopy, and the first screening happens at age 50. Some people may need to have colon cancer screening earlier than age 50 if there is a history of colon cancer in the family.

Oral cancer screening is done by a dentist. It is important to see a dentist to check your mouth for any signs of oral cancer. Oral cancer usually appears as a red or white lesion, but oral cancer is hard to find yourself. Be sure to see your dentist every 6 months for regular checkups, which includes an examination of the mouth, not just the teeth.

TESTOSTERONE AND HIV

Testosterone is the primary male hormone. About 20% of men who are living with HIV have low testosterone levels. The normal testosterone level for men is between 300 and 1,200. Having a low testosterone level can result in symptoms that include having less energy, feeling "down" or depressed, and having less interest in sex (low sex drive). You can have your testosterone level checked through a simple blood test. If you do have a low testosterone level, testosterone can be supplemented with prescription medication in the form of injections, a patch, or a gel. If you have questions about testosterone, talk to your healthcare provider.

Tips for preventing infections

1. In addition to preventing diseases and cancers, it is important for everyone to prevent infections like colds and flu and skin infections too. Here are some tips that you can use to help prevent infections. Encourage those around you to do these too

2. Wash your hands. The important role of washing your hands with soap and water before eating, before and after handling food (cooking), and after using the bathroom cannot be overemphasized

3. Carry antibacterial hand gel. Using these hand gels, which are now available just about everywhere, is just as effective in preventing infection as washing your hands. Of course, hand gels do not remove dirt, but as far as reducing germs, they work just as well

4. Do the vampire cough. Instead of coughing or sneezing into your hand (and then accidently touching something or someone with your hands before you can wash them), do the vampire cough. Raise your forearm and cough or sneeze into the fold of your forearm

5. You need good nutrition. Eating a healthy diet is important to keep your immune system healthy so it can fight off infections

6. Get enough sleep. Sleep is very important for all aspects of good health, not just preventing infection. Be sure that you get enough sleep every day

7. Take care of your teeth. Healthy teeth are very important in the prevention of infection. Dental caries and decay (cavities) can be a source of serious infections of the skin, heart, and brain. Have a dental checkup every 6 months, brush your teeth at least twice a day, and use dental floss at least twice a day. Change your toothbrush often to prevent germs from building up on the toothbrush

Get Up To Date on Vaccines

It is recommended that people living with HIV have hepatitis A and B vaccines. Hepatitis vaccines are usually given just once in your lifetime. Sometimes people who have HIV need a hepatitis vaccine booster. People living with HIV should have an influenza (flu) vaccine every year. Pneumovax (pneumonia) vaccine is also recommended for people living with HIV. The pneumonia vaccine is given at baseline, then again in 5 years. You just need two pneumonia vaccines in a lifetime.

What Nurses Know ...

People with HIV should AVOID live vaccines including shingles, smallpox, and anthrax.

Tips for staying healthy

o At the end of the book is a sheet providing health tips for men; there also is a summary of everything in this chapter plus a few other helpful hints about wellness and prevention that are discussed in other parts of the book. This information is important for all men—not just men who are living with HIV.

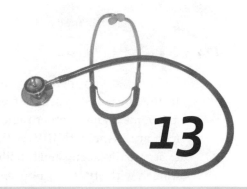

13

Women's Health

I have hot flashes and night sweats ... Is my viral load out of control ... do I have AIDS?   SYLVIA, AGE 51

My periods are irregular ... Is it from my HIV?   JANESSA, AGE 19

Neither of these women's symptoms are from HIV or AIDS. They are just a part of being a woman. Women in their 50s who are experiencing menopause often have hot flashes and night sweats. Many young women have irregular periods. But the first thing Sylvia and Janessa thought was that something must be wrong with their HIV disease.

What we have noticed, after many years of taking care of women who are living with HIV, is that no matter what the symptom, the first thing a woman who is living with HIV thinks and fears—even if its as simple as the common cold—is that the symptoms may be related to their HIV and something is wrong. This is especially true early on for the first few years after being diagnosed with HIV.

There are an increasing number of women living with HIV. In the United States, about 27% of the people living with HIV are women, and in other regions of the world more women than men are living with HIV. With treatment, women with HIV can expect to live a long and full life. The latest predictions show that women with HIV have a life expectancy that is just 10 years less than women who do not have HIV. The average life expectancy for a woman living in the United States is about 80 years, which means that for women with HIV the life expectancy is about 70 years. Of course, life expectancy varies and depends on many factors such as other health problems, family history, lifestyle, and eating habits.

Women living with HIV experience the same health concerns, health risks, and health issues as any other women. Given that HIV is a chronic manageable illness and that women with HIV can expect to live at least to the age of 70, women with HIV must think about all aspects of their health, including HIV, but not just focus on their HIV infection alone. This chapter reviews general women's health issues that are important for all women, with caveats that are specific to women who are living with HIV.

Now that we have excellent treatment for HIV, most women living with HIV who are doing well with their antiretroviral (ARV) treatment and who do experience health problems need to start thinking about the fact that a lot of the time the problems are likely not related to HIV. The health problems that we now see in people living with HIV disease who are on ARV treatment, have a suppressed (undetectable) viral load, and have a high CD4 cell count (over 300) most often occur for other reasons. So, again, while it is very important to pay attention to your HIV, CD4 cell count, and viral load, it is just as important to pay attention to the rest of your body (and mind) too.

Many of the things that threaten women's health are preventable. The Centers for Disease Control has complied data about the seven top causes for poor health among all women. This chapter focuses on those top causes and provides strategies and "tips" to prevent them, and provides information about many other important women's health issues. You will soon see that many of these tips are the same for a lot of women's health risks that are discussed in this chapter. As you are reading, remember that the key to good health is to stay on top of your health—it is the best way to keep it!

The Top Seven Health Problems among Women

HEART DISEASE

Heart disease has often been thought of as a disease of men. The truth is, it is also a major health problem for women. Here are some things you can do to lower your risk for heart disease.

Do not smoke. If you do smoke (or use other tobacco products, like chewing or smoking cigars), ask your healthcare providers about programs and medicines that can help you quit. Remember that secondhand smoke is just as harmful so avoid being in places where people are smoking or being around others while they smoke.

Choose healthy foods. Eat plenty of vegetables and fruits (fresh or frozen), whole grains, high-fiber foods, and lean sources of protein, such as fish. Limit foods high in saturated fat and sodium. This does not mean you can not have the occasional cookie or piece of pie, but most of the time you should eat healthy foods.

Take care of health problems that can cause heart disease. Get your cholesterol and blood pressure checked at least every 6 months. If you know you have high cholesterol or high blood pressure, be sure to keep those controlled with lifestyle changes (healthy eating, exercise) and with medications (if needed). If you have diabetes, keep your blood sugar under control.

Stay active. Include physical activity in your daily routine. Choose sports or other activities you enjoy. Fast walking and dancing are great forms of exercise, and you do not even have to go to the gym.

Control your weight. Those extra pounds increase the risk of heart disease.

Limit alcohol. If you choose to drink alcohol, do so only in moderation. Too much alcohol can raise your blood pressure, which in turn can cause heart disease.

Manage stress. If you constantly worry or are on edge, take steps to reduce stressor learn to deal with stress in healthy ways. Talk to your healthcare providers about programs and treatments that are available to help with stress. If you cannot change the things in your life that cause stress, then consider yoga or another healthy form of stress relief to help deal with the stress.

CANCER

There are several types of cancers that are of concern to women. To reduce the risk of cancer in general, here are some tips.

Do not smoke. Remember, using any type of tobacco puts you at risk for cancer. Avoid secondhand smoke; it counts too.

Maintain a healthy weight. Losing those extra pounds—and keeping them off—may lower the risk of several types of cancer.

Get moving. Exercise/physical activity on its own may lower the risk of certain types of cancer. It will also help you lose those extra pounds. Even small changes can help—do not park in the closest spot to the door, walk to close places instead of driving or taking the bus, and take the stairs instead of the elevator.

Eat fruits and veggies. It may help reduce your risk for cancer.

Protect your skin from the sun. We all need some sun, but a sunburn or prolonged sun exposure is not good for our skin. So, when you are outdoors, cover up and use plenty of sunscreen.

Limit alcohol. Alcohol can increase the risk for several types of cancer—cancer of the breast, colon, lung, kidney, and liver. The risk increases with the amount of alcohol you drink and the length of time you have been drinking regularly. If you choose to drink alcohol, do it in moderation.

Get routine cancer screenings. Be sure to get regular mammograms and other cancer screenings like Pap tests, colonoscopies, and anal cancer screenings.

STROKE

There are some risk factors for stroke that cannot be controlled. These include your family history, age, and race, but there are quite a few others that you can control.

Cholesterol, blood pressure, and blood sugar. Be sure you know what your cholesterol, blood pressure, and blood sugar levels are. If you have high cholesterol (hyperlipidemia), high blood pressure (hypertension), or high blood sugar (diabetes), get them treated and keep them under control.

Do not smoke. If you do smoke, ask for help so you can quit.

Eat a healthy diet. Limit foods high in saturated fat and cholesterol (like greasy, fatty, fried foods).

Keep moving. Include physical activity in your daily routine. If you are overweight, start working on losing those extra pounds.

Limit alcohol. If you choose to drink alcohol, drink in moderation—for women, that means no more than one drink per day.

CHRONIC LUNG DISEASES

Another type of disease that has in the past been associated with men is chronic lung disease. But these diseases, which include bronchitis and emphysema, also are a concern for women. To protect your lungs, here are some tips.

Do not smoke. If you do smoke, ask for help so you can you quit. Also avoid exposure to secondhand smoke.

Stay away from pollution. Stay away from exposure to chemicals and outdoor air pollution.

Prevent lung infections. Wash your hands often. Get vaccinated for flu (every year) and pneumonia (given twice, once at baseline and then a second one 5 years later).

ALZHEIMER'S DISEASE

There is no proven way to prevent Alzheimer's disease, but here are some steps that are thought to perhaps help.

Blood pressure, cholesterol, heart health, and blood sugar. Health problems like high blood pressure, high cholesterol, heart disease, stroke, and diabetes may increase the risk of developing Alzheimer's. Keep these health problems under control by making sure you know your blood pressure, cholesterol, and blood sugar levels. If you do have these health problems, keep them controlled through healthy lifestyle and medications, if needed.

Do not smoke. Some research has suggested a link between smoking and Alzheimer's.

Be active every day. Any movement counts.

Stay mentally and socially active. Practice mental exercises like crossword puzzles. Learn new things, like a new language. Have contact with other people.

ACCIDENTS

Car accidents are a leading cause of death among women. Stay safe on the road and use common sense. Wear your seat belt! Follow the speed limit. Do not drive while under the influence of alcohol or any other drugs and when feeling sleepy. And please, do not text or talk on your cell phone while driving.

TYPE 2 DIABETES

There are two types of diabetes: type 1 and type 2 diabetes. Type 1 is the diabetes of childhood and usually occurs in young children. Type 2 diabetes is the most common type of diabetes and usually starts in adulthood, but it can start in children later in their preteen and teen years.

Type 2 diabetes is a health problem that affects the way your body processes and uses blood sugar (glucose). High levels of blood sugar (poorly controlled diabetes) can lead to heart disease, eye problems (including blindness), nerve damage (diabetic neuropathy), and kidney problems (including kidney failure).

To prevent type 2 diabetes, get serious about your eating and lifestyle habits. Eat healthy and exercise and lose those extra pounds.

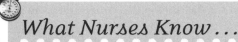

What Nurses Know...

It is hard to change lifestyle habits, but do not feel intimidated. Instead, do whatever you can to lead a healthy lifestyle. Start with small steps; instead of drinking soda every day with lunch, start drinking water. Instead of taking the closest parking spot to the front door, choose a spot that is a little farther away and walk a few extra steps—those types of small steps will lead to bigger steps. Simple preventive measures can go a long way toward reducing your health risks.

Women-Specific Health Issues

BREAST CANCER

While men can get breast cancer, most breast cancer occurs in women. According to the National Cancer Institute, about 12% of women born in the United States (about 1 in 8) will develop breast cancer at some point in her life. HIV in and of itself does not increase the risk for breast cancer.

Breasts contain tissues of varying consistency. Glandular tissue—primarily felt in the upper, outer part of the breast—usually feels firm and slightly rope-like, bumpy or lumpy (nodular). Surrounding fat tissue—often felt in the inner and lower parts of the breast—is soft. You may find that breast-related symptoms, such as tenderness or lumpiness, differ over the course of your menstrual cycle. Breast tissue also changes as you age, typically becoming more fatty and less dense over time.

If you find a breast lump or other change in your breast, you may be worried about breast cancer—but do not panic. The odds are in your favor. Most (four out of five breast lumps) that are biopsied turn out to be noncancerous (benign). However, it is very important to have any breast lump evaluated by a healthcare provider. If you need help finding a breast health provider, ask your HIV healthcare provider. Another place to find help is by contacting your local Komen for the Cure affiliate or your local American Cancer Society chapter.

It is important to be familiar with how your breasts normally feel, thus if there is a change in your breasts, you will know it. These are reasons that you should see a healthcare provider about your breasts:

- You find a breast lump that is new or unusual and feels different from the way your breast usually feels
- A new breast lump does not go away after your next period
- A breast lump seems to have changed—it gets bigger
- Bloody discharge from your nipple
- Skin changes on your breast, like redness, crusting, dimpling, or puckering
- Your nipple suddenly turns inward (inversion)

Mammograms

A mammogram is an image of your breast and it is used to screen for breast cancer. Mammograms are key in detecting breast cancer early, and mammograms help decrease breast cancer deaths.

During a mammogram, your breasts are compressed between two firm surfaces to spread out the breast tissue. Then, a machine captures images of your breasts that a physician specialist (radiologist) looks at and determines if any changes or cancer is seen.

A mammogram can be used for either screening or diagnosis. How often you should have a mammogram depends on your age and your risk of breast cancer. Women who have a history of a first-degree relative (mother, sister, aunt, grandmother) who had breast cancer prior to menopause are at a higher risk for breast cancer and should have mammograms starting early in their life. If you are a woman who has a first-degree relative who had breast cancer (at any age), you need to let your healthcare provider know. For women who do not have a family history of breast cancer, there is some controversy about when to have the first mammogram, but most experts agree that it should be between age 40 and 50. Most women without a family history of breast cancer have their first screening mammogram at age 40.

CERVICAL CANCER

The cervix (the lower part of the uterus that connects to the vagina) is the location where cervical cancer occurs. Almost all cervical cancers are caused by human papillomavirus (HPV), a sexually transmitted infection.

Most of the time, when exposed to HPV, a woman's immune system prevents HPV from doing harm. However, in some women, HPV survives for years and contributes to a process that causes the cells on the surface of the cervix to become cancer cells. In the United States and many other countries, the death rate from cervical cancer has dropped significantly. This drop is due, in large part, to cervical cancer screening with Pap testing.

There is now a vaccine to prevent HPV infection. It is recommended that young women and men get vaccinated for HPV prior to becoming sexually active. Widespread HPV vaccination could lead to even lower rates of cervical cancer, or even elimination.

Pap smear

A Pap smear, also called a Pap test, is a screening procedure to test for cervical cancer in women. A Pap smear involves collecting cells from the cervix. Early detection of cervical cancer with a Pap smear gives you a greater chance at a cure. A Pap smear can also detect changes in your cervical cells that suggest cancer may develop in the future. Detecting these cells early with a Pap smear is the first step in stopping the development of cervical cancer in the future.

Colposcopy

A colposcopy is a procedure that examines the cervix, vagina, and vulva for signs of disease using an instrument called a colposcope. A colposcopy is recommended when a Pap test shows abnormal results. For women who have HIV disease, any abnormal Pap test is followed by a colposcopy. During colposcopy, a sample of tissue (biopsy) is usually collected and sent for further laboratory testing. If you have an abnormal Pap and are asked to have a colposcopy, this does not necessarily mean you have cancer. But it is important to follow abnormal Pap tests with colposcopy because detecting abnormal cells, or cancer cells, early on results in the best chance to stop cancer from developing or to cure the cancer.

Many women experience anxiety before their colposcopy exams. Knowing what to expect during your colposcopy may help you feel more comfortable. Before you have a colposcopy, ask your healthcare provider to explain the procedure to you step by step. Colposcopy is a procedure that is done in the office (outpatient) setting and does not require anesthesia. You can drive yourself to/from the colposcopy appointment.

YOUR MENSTRUAL CYCLE

Each month a woman's body goes through a series of changes to prepare for the possibility of a pregnancy. Every month, one of a woman's two ovaries releases an egg—a process called "ovulation." At the same time, there are changes in the female hormones that prepare the uterus for pregnancy. If ovulation takes place and the egg is not fertilized (the woman does not become pregnant), then the lining of the uterus sheds through the vagina, called a menstrual period (menstrual flow).

A menstrual cycle starts on the first day of one period to the first day of the next, and this cycle is not the same for every woman. Menstrual flow may occur every 21 to 35 days and last 2 to 7 days. For the first few years after menstruation begins, long cycles are common. However, menstrual cycles tend to shorten and become more regular as women get older. Your menstrual cycle may be regular—about the same length every month—or somewhat irregular, and your period (menstrual flow) may be light or heavy, painful or pain-free, long or short. All of these are considered normal. There is a broad range of normal and it is important to know what is normal for you.

Do you know when your last menstrual period began or how long it lasted? If not, it might be time to start paying attention. Tracking your menstrual cycles and timing ovulation can help you understand what is normal for you and identify important changes—such as a missed period or unpredictable menstrual bleeding. While menstrual cycle irregularities usually are not serious, sometimes they can signal health problems.

HIV does not usually interfere with a woman's menstrual cycles. However, if a woman has an advanced HIV disease (AIDS) or an opportunistic infection, the menstrual cycle can stop. Most of the time, once ARV therapy is started and the woman's immune system improves, then her menstrual cycles become normal again.

To find out what is normal for your menstrual cycle, start keeping a record of your menstrual cycle. Track your start date every month for several months in a row on a calendar. Write down any problems or concerns you may have about the timing, flow, or discomfort of your periods. Also write down the end date, the type of flow (light/heavy), and any pain. Menstrual cycle irregularities can have many different causes; here are some of the most common.

Pregnancy. A delayed or missed period can be an early sign of pregnancy. If you have not had your period in 6 weeks and you have been sexually active, take a pregnancy test.

Eating disorders, extreme weight loss, or excessive exercising can disrupt menstruation.

Polycystic ovary syndrome. This is a common hormonal disorder that can cause small cysts to develop in the ovaries together with irregular periods.

Endometriosis. This disorder causes tissue that normally lines the inside of your uterus to grow outside your uterus. It can cause pain, especially during your period.

Pelvic inflammatory disease. This infection of the reproductive organs may cause irregular menstrual bleeding.

Fibroids. Uterine fibroids are noncancerous growths of the uterus. They may cause heavy menstrual periods and bleeding between periods.

You should contact a healthcare provider about your menstrual cycle if you experience

- Menstrual periods that suddenly stop for more than 90 days
- Menstrual periods that become erratic after having been regular
- Bleeding for more than 7 days
- Heavy bleeding that is more than usual, soaking through more the one pad or tampon every 1 to 2 hours
- Periods that are less than 21 days or more than 35 days apart
- Bleeding between periods
- Severe pain during your period
- Fever and feeling sick after using tampons

Menopause

Menopause is the permanent end of menstruation and fertility, defined as occurring 12 months after your last menstrual period. Menopause is a natural process, not an illness. However, the changes that occur during menopause can cause physical and emotional symptoms that can disrupt sleep, cause fatigue, and sometimes cause feelings of sadness and loss. Even though menopause is not a disease, a woman should not hesitate to seek

What Nurses Know . . .

For more information about menopause, we highly recommend the book What Nurses Know ... Menopause *by Karen Roush. The book is excellent and provides the answers to almost any question about menopause. Remember, menopause is a normal part of a woman's life, and a woman with HIV who is aging typically goes through menopause just like all other women who are aging.*

treatment for severe symptoms of menopause. There are effective treatments that are available to help.

OTHER CANCER SCREENINGS

Colon cancer screening. There are several tests available to screen for colon cancer. The most common screening test is called "colonoscopy," and the first screening happens at age 50. Some people may need to have colon cancer screening earlier than age 50 if there is a history of colon cancer in the family.

Anal cancer screening. Screening for anal cancer is pretty new. Anal cancer is much more common in individuals who are living with HIV. While it is more common in men who have sex with men, anal cancer occurs in women too. Anal cancer, like cervical cancer, is caused by HPV. Anal Pap testing and high-resolution anoscopy are the two screening tests available for anal cancer. Women living with HIV should be screened for anal cancer once a year.

Oral cancer screening. This type of screening is done by a dentist. It is important to see a dentist to check your mouth for any signs of oral cancer. Oral cancer usually appears as a red or white lesion, but oral cancer is hard to find yourself. Be sure to see your dentist every 6 months for regular checkups, which includes an examination of the mouth, not just the teeth.

Tips for preventing infections

In addition to preventing diseases and cancers, it is important for everyone to prevent infections like colds and flu and skin infections too. Here are some tips that you can use to help prevent infections. Encourage those around you to do these too.

o Wash your hands. The important role of washing your hands with soap and water before eating, before and after handling food (cooking), and after using the bathroom cannot be overemphasized. This behavior in and of itself will greatly protect you and others from spreading, and catching, infections

○ Carry antibacterial hand gel. Using these hand gels, which are now available just about everywhere, is just as effective in preventing infection as washing your hands. Of course, hand gels do not remove dirt, but as far as reducing germs they work just as well

○ Do the vampire cough. Instead of coughing or sneezing into your hand (and then accidently touching something or someone with your hands before you can wash them), do the vampire cough. Raise your forearm and cough or sneeze into the fold of your forearm

○ You need good nutrition. Eating a healthy diet is important to keep your immune system healthy so it can fight off infections. Balance the amount of calories you need over three meals a day plus two snacks and make sure you are eating a balance of foods that are high in protein and low in fats, and be sure to include plenty of fruits and vegetables. Keep salty, fatty, processed, and sugary foods to a minimum

○ Get enough sleep. Sleep is very important for all aspects of good health, not just preventing infection. Be sure that you get enough sleep every day. If you have problems getting good sleep, here are what sleep experts can help: go to bed at the same time every day and get up at the same time every day, avoid caffeine and alcohol for several hours before going to bed, use your bed only for sleeping or sex (do not use your bed to watch TV or to read), if you cannot get to sleep then do not just lay in bed—do something like reading a book in your living room—then go back to bed when you feel sleepy

○ Take care of your teeth. Healthy teeth are very important in the prevention of infection. Dental caries and decay (cavities) can be a source of serious infections of the skin, heart, and brain. Have a dental checkup every 6 months, brush your teeth at least twice a day, and use dental floss at least twice a day. Change your toothbrush often to prevent germs from building up on the toothbrush

Get Up To Date on Vaccines

It is recommended that people living with HIV have hepatitis A and B vaccines. Hepatitis vaccines are usually given just once in your lifetime. Sometimes people who have HIV need a hepatitis vaccine booster. People living with HIV should have an influenza (flu) vaccine every year. Pneumovax (pneumonia) vaccine is also recommended for people living with HIV. The pneumonia vaccine is given at baseline, then again in 5 years. You just need two pneumonia vaccines in a lifetime.

What Nurses Know . . .

People with HIV should AVOID shingles, smallpox, and anthrax vaccines.

Tips for staying healthy

○ There is a sheet on women's health at the end of the book. You may want to make copies of this summary and give it as a handout to women in your life. This information is important for all women—not just women who are living with HIV.

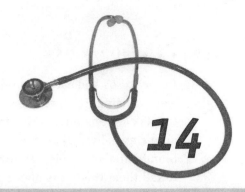

14

Having a Family

My husband and I were really excited when I found out I was pregnant. I had been sick with flu-like symptoms for a few weeks and then I went to a clinic for a checkup. The doctor told me the good news that I was pregnant, but then she called in a counselor and together they told me there was more news. I had tested positive for HIV. HIV was one of the routine tests I'd had as part of my prenatal testing. I was so scared. I was so afraid my baby would have HIV too. I was told there was treatment to prevent transmission of HIV from mother to baby and that the treatment was about 99% effective.

I thank God every day that I was diagnosed with HIV early and that I was given ARV medications during my pregnancy for my own health and to prevent transmission of HIV to my baby. I had to give my baby liquid AZT for the first 6 weeks of her life. She did not get HIV. Today, my daughter is beautiful and healthy and she is just about to start kindergarten. My husband did not have HIV and to this day he remains HIV negative. We are now trying to have another baby and we will keep my husband HIV negative with the help of God and the help of healthcare providers who are specialists in pregnancy and HIV. SARAH, AGE 29

In the 1980s and early to mid-1990s, most healthcare providers were advising HIV-infected women not to have babies because of the risk of transmitting HIV to the fetus (baby) during pregnancy or during delivery. For the women who did get pregnant—or who found out about their HIV diagnosis during pregnancy—we had to tell them there was about a 30% to 40% risk that their baby could be born with HIV. It was terrible. Back then, we did not know much about how babies became HIV infected during pregnancy, let alone how to prevent vertical transmission of HIV (i.e., mother passing HIV to her baby). Also the young HIV-infected women were devastated about the fact that they could never have children. I clearly remember one young woman in my community who in the late 1990s made an HIV prevention video. In the video, she advised women to protect their sexual health and she stated: "If you get HIV you can never have children … I always thought I'd have children … my dog is my baby now." We have lost track of that woman, but have often wondered if now, in the 21st century, she has been able to have a family.

Today, a conversation about pregnancy with a woman, or couple, who is living with HIV is a totally different conversation. We now have the knowledge, skills, and medications to help women who are living with HIV have a healthy (HIV-negative) baby, if that is what the woman wants. We have photos in our offices of the many healthy babies that have been born to HIV-infected women we have taken care of during their pregnancies. Things have really changed when it comes to HIV and pregnancy in the last 20 years!

This chapter focuses on the issues of HIV and pregnancy. This chapter is not about pregnancy care itself. If you are pregnant and want specific information about prenatal care, pregnancy, and/or delivery, ask your women's healthcare provider for a referral to a good source of information about pregnancy.

Women with HIV disease who are pregnant are considered high risk during their pregnancy. If you have HIV and are pregnant, you should seek care from a team of health experts who are experienced at taking care of pregnant women living with HIV.

Also make sure the hospital where you plan to deliver your baby has experience in this area of healthcare. There is evidence to support the fact that receiving care from healthcare providers and hospitals that are experienced in both pregnancy and HIV leads to the best outcomes.

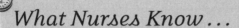

What Nurses Know . . .

Women with HIV who are pregnant should receive care by a team of healthcare providers, including an HIV specialist who has experience treating women with HIV during pregnancy and a women's health specialist who has experience taking care of pregnant women with HIV disease.

HIV Testing in Pregnancy

Since 2002, the Centers for Disease Control has recommended that all pregnant women be routinely screened for HIV infection in the first trimester of pregnancy. Repeat HIV testing in the third trimester of pregnancy is recommended by the American College of Obstetricians and Gynecologists in areas where there is a high HIV prevalence among women of child-bearing age. In routine healthcare practice, many healthcare providers and hospitals have adopted routine HIV testing both in the first and third trimesters of pregnancy.

Identifying HIV infection during pregnancy is very important because perinatal (from mother to baby) HIV transmission is preventable. In the United States, the current standard treatment to prevent mother-to-baby HIV transmission includes starting antiretroviral (ARV) therapy on the mother during the second trimester, giving the mother intravenous azidothymidine (AZT) or zidovudine during the delivery, giving the baby liquid AZT for the first 6 weeks of life, and avoiding breast-feeding. With this protocol, the transmission rate from mother to baby can be reduced to less than 1%.

HIV and Pregnancy Scenarios

Due to aggressive screening of pregnant women and ready access to ARV therapy, a very small number of children are born HIV infected in the United States. Most children born to HIV-infected mothers are healthy and are not infected with HIV. The number of HIV-infected women having children is increasing. There are several reasons for the growing number. First, there is a high percentage of HIV-infected U.S. women who desire and intend to have children, and there are more women being identified and diagnosed with HIV infection during prenatal care. Finally, HIV-infected women who have had a healthy child often want to have more children.

There are four common scenarios that we see in our practice with regard to HIV and pregnancy.

1. Mother has HIV and plans the pregnancy
2. Mother is diagnosed with HIV early during her prenatal care screenings
3. Mother is diagnosed with HIV at the third trimester or at delivery
4. Mother is not screened for HIV at any time during her pregnancy or delivery and is diagnosed after the baby is born

Obviously, the first scenario is the best one. If a woman living with HIV decides to have a baby, seeks prenatal counseling, and plans the pregnancy together with her family and her healthcare providers, this leads to the best chances of a good outcome. The second scenario, while it can be a very emotional pregnancy due to the new diagnosis of HIV, usually can result in a good outcome for the baby and the baby is born healthy and free of HIV. Also, in the second scenario the mother has been diagnosed early in her HIV disease and this affords the mother an excellent prognosis for her own HIV disease. Even with the third scenario, there are still ARV treatment interventions at the end of the pregnancy and during the delivery that can be implemented to prevent transmission of HIV from the mother to the baby. Also with the third scenario, there is still the opportunity to give the baby oral liquid AZT for the first 6 weeks of life, further reducing the risk for transmission of HIV to the baby.

The fourth scenario is the one with the most risk for the baby acquiring HIV. Unfortunately, even with aggressive screening and treatment, there are some mothers who are not tested or treated for HIV during pregnancy. This scenario is especially true for developing countries with limited resources. Sadly, the highest number of children born HIV-infected live in poor countries. Despite aggressive HIV screening among pregnant women in the United States, there are still babies born every year with HIV infection: about one or two babies are born HIV-infected per state each year.

What Nurses Know . . .

Pregnancy can be a very emotional time in a woman's life. For a woman who has HIV and is pregnant, it can be a particularly stressful time. Stress can be even higher if the pregnancy was unplanned or if the diagnosis of HIV was made during the pregnancy. Remember that help is available. If you need help dealing with the emotional or physical stress of pregnancy and/or coping with the diagnosis of HIV, talk to someone about it that you trust, such as your healthcare provider or your case manager.

Children and HIV

Children with HIV are a vulnerable population. For children who are born HIV infected, there is the prospect of lifelong ARV treatment together with the stigma of having HIV. In addition, all children (HIV infected and those who are not HIV infected) whose parents have HIV disease are at higher risk for developmental, social, economic, and psychological problems related to their parents' HIV status. Research indicates that children with HIV face greater challenges to their psychosocial well-being, that is their mental health and quality of life. Some of the problems that children with HIV can experience are complex and they are complicated by their parents' own ability to deal with HIV. Among the problems are isolation, loss of their childhood, reduced access to social programs, and financial stress. The health status of the mother, and the father, directly impacts the child(ren)'s psychosocial health. If the mother has depression or if mother/father are chronically ill adults, then this increases the risk for poor psychosocial outcomes for the child(ren).

Very little research has been conducted to understand the relationship between HIV, motherhood, and outcomes for infants and children. The research that has been done indicates that the following strategies may improve the outcomes for children who have HIV-infected mothers/fathers. Intervention programs that focus on the mothers living with HIV have been found to be helpful. Such interventions include in-home visits by nurses and group interventions to help mothers with coping skills. There are also several intervention programs that have been developed that target HIV-infected children, especially in countries with high numbers of children who are living with HIV.

Disclosure of HIV Status and Children

The decision by a mother, a father, or both about whether to disclose his/her/their HIV status to his/her/their child(ren) can be difficult. Once that decision has been made, then the next question is when and how to disclose such information, which can be very difficult. Also, the decision about when to tell a child that he or she has HIV infection is also very difficult. These decisions are very personal in nature, and each family must decide what is best for them.

There is help available to families who want and need to make these decisions. If you are a parent who is living with HIV and you are struggling with the decision about whether or what to tell your child(ren) about HIV, get help. Ask your healthcare provider or your case manager for a referral to an agency or a counselor who can help you decide if, how, and when to disclose information about your HIV status or your child's HIV status. You may also want to talk to other parents who are living with HIV and have been or are in your same situation. Many communities have support groups for people who are living with HIV and such groups can be very helpful when one is struggling with these types of decisions.

Two Moms, Two Dads, and Discordant Couples

Most of this chapter has focused on the scenario of HIV and pregnancy when the woman who is carrying the child is the one who is infected with HIV. But what about other family situations like two moms, two dads, or discordant couples? In all of these cases, a couple living with HIV can opt to have a family if they want to. While there are no guarantees when it comes to making a baby, with the right help, the odds for a successful pregnancy and a healthy baby are good.

TWO MOMS

The options for same-gender female couples vary, depending on the HIV status of the partners. If one woman in the couple is HIV negative and has no other health problems that would keep her from having a healthly pregnancy, then she is likely the best choice for carrying a baby. If both women have HIV disease and one of them wants to have the baby, then the treatment scenario is the same as what we have described earlier in this chapter for HIV-infected pregnant women. In either case, a sperm donor would be utilized.

Another option for a same-gender couple, or for any couple who is having fertility problems, is a surrogate mother. And remember, there is always adoption. Now that people with HIV are living long and have healthy life spans, there is really no health-related reason that we can think of for why a person with HIV should not consider adoption.

For more information about fertility options that are available to same-gender couples, or any couple having fertility problems, see a women's health specialist, an infertility specialist, or a reproductive endocrinologist. Ask your healthcare provider to give you a referral to a reputable physician in your community.

TWO DADS

Same-gender male couples who are living with HIV may also opt for the family life. Options for same-gender male couples include using a surrogate mother. If one of the men wants to be the sperm donor for a surrogate, there is a technique known as "sperm washing" that can remove HIV from sperm and make it safe to use for purposes of pregnancy. Again, adoption is an option too.

DISCORDANT COUPLES

For male/female couples who are discordant (one is HIV infected and the other is not), the options for having a family vary, depending on which partner is HIV infected. In the case of a woman who is HIV infected and wants to become pregnant, the man's sperm can be introduced into her vagina using a device, instead of the couple having unprotected intercourse. This "assisted" insemination will protect the man from risk of HIV infection. Engaging the help of a healthcare provider who is a specialist in pregnancy is very important, as the timing of when to introduce the sperm is critical for a successful pregnancy in these cases. If you are in this situation, ask your HIV healthcare provider for a referral to a women's health specialist or to an infertility specialist who is experienced in HIV and pregnancy.

In the case of a man who is HIV positive and wants to have a baby with a woman who is HIV negative, sperm washing is the safest way to ensure that the woman does not become HIV infected. Again, it is important to plan such a pregnancy with the help of a healthcare provider who is experienced in HIV and pregnancy.

We know that most pregnancies are unplanned. But in the case of HIV, regardless of which scenario you are in, it is best to engage in family planning in advance. If you are thinking about having a baby, or adopting a baby, talk to a healthcare provider before you become pregnant or go to an adoption agency. Planning in advance and talking with a healthcare provider, or healthcare providers, who have experience in family planning, HIV, and pregnancy gives you the best chance for a successful pregnancy, delivery, or adoption of a healthy child.

Glossary

Adherence: Act of "sticking to something." Like making a decision to take all of your medications without missing a dose.

AIDS: Stands for acquired immune deficiency syndrome and is late-stage HIV infection. AIDS occurs when a person who has HIV has a CD4 cell count less than 200 or is diagnosed with certain cancers or *opportunistic infections*.

Anemia: Loss of red blood cells. Red blood cells are necessary to take oxygen to all parts of the body.

Anorexia: Loss of appetite. Having anorexia for an extended period of time could lead to weight loss. Anorexia can be caused by many factors including depression, HIV, or medications.

Antibiotic: Drug that kills or slows the growth of bacteria (organisms that cause infection). Penicillin is an example of a widely used antibiotic.

Antifungal: Drug that kills or slows the growth of a fungus (an organism that can cause infections).

Antigen: Substance that is able to cause antibodies to spread.

Antiretrovirals (ARVs): Medications used to treat HIV. ARVs stop the replication of HIV and reduce the HIV viral load.

Antiviral: Drug or process that kills a virus or suppresses its ability to reproduce.

ART: Stands for antiretroviral therapy, a term used when referring to the combination of drugs a person is taking for treatment of HIV.

Asymptomatic: Absence of, or not having, symptoms. A person may have been infected with HIV for many years but does not have any symptoms of the infection; their disease is described as asymptomatic.

Bacteria: Tiny organisms that may cause illness, such as diarrhea or pneumonia.

Baseline: Term used to describe a person's condition or lab measurements when first diagnosed, or before starting medications.

Biopsy: Removal of a small amount of tissue to examine for evidence of certain cancers or diseases. A biopsy may be done in a provider's office or clinic. A more invasive biopsy may need to be done in an operating room.

Blood count: Also known as CBC, this refers to tests done to measure the size, number, and structure of white blood cells, red blood cells, and platelets in the blood.

Blood gases: A test that shows how well the lungs are working.

Bone marrow: Soft tissue inside the bone where the production of blood cells takes place.

Bronchoscopy: A procedure using an instrument (a bronchoscope) to look at the lung passages. The bronchoscope, a tube-like instrument, is passed through the patient's nose or mouth and down into the airway. The doctor is able to look inside the lungs and obtain tissue samples to help in diagnosing the patient's illness.

Candida: A type of fungal infection that is often an early warning sign of HIV. Oral *Candida,* often called thrush, infects the mouth with small whitish patches that can be painful and cause difficulty swallowing. Thrush can spread to the esophagus and make eating solid foods painful. Vaginal candidiasis is a serious health problem in HIV-infected women.

CAT scan or CT scan: A special x-ray where organs can simultaneously be x-rayed at multiple angles.

CD4 count: Also called CD4 cell or T4 cell count. It is the measure of the number of CD4 cells in the blood. CD4 cells are white blood cells that HIV selectively infects and destroys. Having an adequate number of CD4 cells is vital for normal immune functions.

CDC: Stands for Centers for Disease Control and Prevention. A federal health agency that monitors and investigates diseases such as HIV.

Chronic: Lasting a long time or recurring.

Clinical trial: A study of an experimental drug in human subjects, which takes place in a hospital or clinic.

Colonoscopy: Procedure using a lighted, flexible tube to examine the large bowel.

Combination therapy: The use of two or more drugs to fight HIV or other infections.

Cryptococcosis: An infectious disease seen in patients with HIV. It is acquired through the respiratory tract.

Cryptosporidium: An intestinal parasite causing diarrhea, and possibly weight loss.

Dementia: Loss of mental abilities, with symptoms such as confusion, memory loss, and decreased intellectual functioning.

Diagnosis: The process of determining the cause and nature of a person's illness. This is usually done by examining the person's medical history, physical examination, symptoms, and monitoring laboratory tests.

Diarrhea: Unusually frequent, watery, and/or loose stools.

DNA: Deoxyribonucleic acid. A molecule that controls cell reproduction. HIV is able to insert itself into a cell's DNA and use the cell's mechanisms to make more copies of HIV.

Efficacy: How effective or potent a medication is in doing its job.

ELISA: Enzyme-linked immunosorbent assay. An early screening test used to detect antibodies to HIV.

Encephalitis: An inflammation or infection of the brain. Common symptoms are fever, headache, seizure, and difficulty concentrating or thinking.

Esophagus: The tube that carries food from the mouth to the stomach. An inflammation of the esophagus may cause pain or difficulty swallowing. Causes of this inflammation may be *Candida*, herpes simplex, or cytomegalovirus.

Experimental drug: A drug that has not been approved and licensed by the government (FDA) and is being studied for safety and/or efficacy in treating patients with a disease.

Fatigue: Lack of energy; physical exhaustion.

FDA: Food and Drug Administration. A part of the U.S. Department of Health and Human Services responsible for regulating development and licensing of drugs.

HAART: Stands for highly active antiretroviral therapy. Usually HAART refers to at least a three-drug regimen that contains two or more classes of drugs. Now often called ART (antiretroviral therapy).

Hairy leukoplakia: An abnormal condition occurring in immunosuppressed persons. Thick white or hair-like patches are seen on the tongue.

Hematocrit: A measurement of the volume of packed red blood cells in the body.

Hemoglobin: The part of the red blood cell that carries oxygen throughout the body.

Hemophilia: An inherited condition where normal blood clotting is not possible. Hemophiliacs (persons with hemophilia) may require frequent transfusions of a blood product called Factor VIII to assist in clotting. Factor VIII is a concentrate made from the pooled blood of many donors.

Hepatitis: An inflammation, or infection, of the liver, causing fever, abdominal pains, and jaundice (a yellow discoloration of the eyes and/or skin).

Herpes simplex virus: HSV-1 is the virus that causes cold sores or fever blisters on the mouth or face. HSV-2 is the virus that causes sores or blisters in the genital area and anus, which is sexually transmitted. In people with HIV, herpes infections can be more severe and last longer.

Herpes varicella-zoster virus: The virus that causes shingles. Small, painful blisters are noted to follow nerve pathways, usually on one side of the body.

High-risk behaviors: These are things people do that increase their chances of transmitting HIV to someone else or contracting (becoming infected with) HIV. Doing things such as having sex without a condom, having more than one sex partner, or sharing needles to inject drugs are some of the high-risk behaviors that spread HIV.

HIV healthcare provider (HCP): A healthcare provider who has additional training and expertise in the management of HIV disease. Research in North America indicates that medical outcomes are better when a person is treated by an HCP who has expertise in treating HIV disease.

HIV or human immunodeficiency virus: The retrovirus identified as causing AIDS.

HIV positive: Term used to describe a person who has HIV.

HIV viral load or viral load (PCR): A blood test that measures the amount of HIV in the blood.

Hypersensitivity: When someone has an allergic-like reaction to a medicine. It may be severe or life threatening. Symptoms may include rash, difficulty breathing, swollen tongue, or fever.

Immune response: The response or activity of the immune system when it discovers an infection.

Immune system: The body's defense mechanisms that work together to assist the body in fighting disease-causing invaders, such as cancer and bacterial, fungal, parasitic, and viral infections.

Immunity: The response of an individual's immune system to protect the body against a certain infectious organism.

Immunoglobulin: A group of antibodies. Antibodies to certain organisms can be pooled from blood donors with immunity and infused into patients.

Immunosuppression: Weakening of the body's immune system.

Incubation period: The time between the initial infection of a disease and the first symptoms. The incubation period for HIV can be from a few months to possibly several years.

Infusion: The process by which a substance, such as medication, can be given to a patient by injecting it into the bloodstream through a vein. Often called "IV" medication.

Lesion: Any abnormal change detected in tissue that is due to disease or injury.

Lymphocyte: A type of white blood cell that fights infection.

Lymphoma: Malignancy, or cancer, of the lymph nodes.

Macrophage: A type of white cell that "eats" dead cells and invading disease organisms such as viruses and bacteria. Unfortunately, it is unable to "eat" HIV.

Maintenance therapy: Use of treatment or treatments (such as medications) to keep a person's health condition stable.

MRI: Magnetic resonance imaging, which is similar to a CT scan. It can provide information on the form and function of internal organs and tissue.

Mycosis: Any disease caused by fungus.

Myopathy: Abnormal condition or disease of the muscle.

Neuropathy: Pain or tingling in the nerves (usually in the feet and hands).

Neutropenia: A decrease in the number of certain white blood cells, called neutrophils. A person with neutropenia is at very high risk for a serious infection.

Night sweats: Heavy sweating to the point of soaking bed sheets.

Opportunistic infection: Life-threatening infections that occur when the immune system is weakened by HIV. Typically these infections occur when a person has less than 200 CD4 cells.

Pancreatitis: Swelling of the pancreas. May cause severe stomach pains and can be life threatening.

Parasite: A plant or animal that lives, grows, and feeds on or within another living thing.

Pathogen: An organism or substance capable of causing disease.

Perinatal: Occurring in the time period around, during, or just after the birth.

Peripheral neuropathy: See neuropathy.

PGL: Stands for persistent generalized lymphadenopathy. Lymph glands are swollen for a long time (persists), lymphadenopathy can occur throughout the body (generalized).

Platelets: Blood elements that are necessary for normal blood clotting. Many HIV-positive people may develop thrombocytopenia or low platelet counts.

PLWA: Stands for person living with AIDS.

PLWHA: Stands for person living with HIV/AIDS.

Prophylaxis: Treatment given to prevent a disease from occurring or spreading.

PWA: Stands for person with AIDS.

Regimen: This refers to a person's schedule for taking HIV drugs. Usually, a plan is developed that helps a person take their medications at a scheduled time, with or without food. A person with HIV **must** adhere to his/her regimen to control HIV disease.

Remission: The period of time when the signs and symptoms of a disease partially or totally go away. The length of time remission may last varies with each disease and each patient.

Resistance: When a drug becomes less effective against HIV, we say that HIV has become resistant to the drug (usually caused by mutations or changes in HIV's genetic material).

Retrovirus: A virus that is able to take over a cell using an enzyme to help change their RNA into DNA.

RNA: Stands for ribonucleic acid. It is a molecule that helps control what goes on inside the cell. It is unable to make new viruses like DNA.

Ryan White Care Act: A federally sponsored program that provides assistance with medications, outpatient medical care, and social services for people living with HIV in the United States.

Salmonellosis: A common form of food poisoning, with symptoms including nausea, vomiting, abdominal cramps, and diarrhea. This infection is caused by *Salmonella* bacteria.

Seroconversion: The time when a person's antibody status changes from negative to positive.

Side effect: An effect of a drug that is not the desired outcome. Sometimes, a drug is stopped because of its side effects, but other times we wait for them to subside. For example, some drugs might cause sedation the first few days of taking it but then it subsides.

STD or sexually transmitted disease (same as STI or sexually transmitted infection): These are infections that are contagious and can be passed on to another person through sexual contact, including oral, vaginal, or anal sex (e.g, herpes, gonorrhea, syphilis, HIV).

Structured treatment interruption: A defined break in taking anti-HIV medications. This is not a drug holiday. Your healthcare provider decides how long you will stop the medications and when you will restart. This is still being studied and has NOT been proven effective.

Systemic infection: An infection spread throughout the body.

T4: See CD4.

Thrombocytopenia: A condition characterized by low platelet counts (platelets are necessary for normal blood clotting).

Thrush: See *Candida.*

Tolerability: Refers to how bearable the side effects of a medication are. For example, if something gives you chronic diarrhea that is hard to live with, that would be low tolerability. If you only experience a mild headache, then that might be considered good or high tolerability.

Toxicity: Toxicity would be a more severe type of side effect. For example, some drugs put a strain on the liver and make it more difficult for the liver to do its job. This is an example of liver toxicity. Lab tests are done routinely to look for changes in normal functioning or toxicity.

Tuberculin skin test: A test to tell if a person has tuberculosis (TB). TB is a lung infection that people living with HIV may be at risk of acquiring.

Tumor: A swelling or an enlargement; an abnormal mass that may be benign (noncancerous) or malignant (cancerous).

Vaccine: A drug that causes the immune system to produce antibodies to fight an organism that causes disease. These antibodies protect a person from getting the disease in the future.

Viral load: The amount of HIV in a person's blood.

Virus: A tiny living organism that invades cells and causes many diseases that can be transmitted from one person to another, such as cold and flu.

Wasting syndrome: Extreme weight loss (10% or more [unintentional]) of the HIV-positive person's average body weight.

Western blot: A blood test used to detect specific antibodies. Used as a second or confirmatory test for HIV.

White blood cells (leukocytes): They are the body's tools for fighting and preventing infection.

Resources

General HIV Advocacy and Professional Organizations

AIDS Healthcare Foundation
6255 W, Sunset Boulevard, 21st Floor
Los Angeles, CA 90028
Phone: 323-860-5200
Web site: www.aidshealth.org

AIDS Research Alliance
1400 South Grand Avenue
Suite 701
Los Angeles, CA 90015
Phone: 310-358-2423
Fax: 310-358-2431
E-mail: info@aidsresearch.org
Web site: www.aidsresearch.org

American Congress of Obstetricians and Gynecologists
PO Box 96920
Washington, DC, 20090-6920
Phone: 202-638-5577
Web site: www.acog.org

amfAR
120 Wall Street, 13th Floor
New York, NY 10005-3908
Phone: 212-806-1600
Fax: 212-806-1601
Web site: www.amfar.org

Association of Nurses in AIDS Care
3538 Ridgewood Road
Akron, OH 44333
Phone: 1-800-260-6780
Fax: 330-670-0109
E-mail: anac@anacnet.org
Web site: www.nursesinaidscare.org

Balm in Gilead
701 East Franklin Street
Suite 1000
Richmond, VA 23219
Phone: 804-644-2256 or 888-225-6243
Web site: www.balmingilead.org

Black AIDS Institute
1833 West 8th Street
Suite 200
Los Angeles, CA 90057-4920
Phone: 213-353-3610
Fax: 213-989-0181
Web site: www.blackaids.org

Centerlink: The Community of LGBT Centers
PO Box 24490
Fort Lauderdale, FL 33307
Phone: 954-765-6024
Fax: 954-765-6593
E-mail: CenterLink@lgbtcenters.org
Web site: www.lgbtcenters.org

Gay Men's Health Crisis
446 West 33rd Street
New York, NY 10001-2601
Web site: www.gmhc.org

GLBT National Help Center
GLBT National Hotline: 888-843-4564
GLBT Youth National Hotline: 800-246-7743
Web site: www.glnh.org

Infectious Disease Society of America and HIV Medicine
   Association
1300 Wilson Boulevard
Suite 300
Arlington, VA 22209
Phone: 703-299-0200
Fax: 703-299-0204
Web sites: www.idsociety.org and www.hivma.org

National AIDS Treatment Advocacy Project
580 Broadway
Suite 1010
New York, NY 10012
Phone: 212-219-0106 or 888-26-NATAP
Fax: 212-219-8473
E-mail: info@natap.org
Web site: www.natap.org

National Minority AIDS Council
1931 13th Street, N2
Washington, DC 20009-4432
Phone: 202-483-6622
Fax: 202-483-1135
E-mail: communications@nmac.org
Web site: www.nmac.org

Project Inform
1375 Mission Street
San Francisco, CA 94103-2621
Phone: 415-558-8669
HIV Health InfoLine: 800-822-7422 (toll-free) or 415-558-9051
    (San Francisco Bay Area/international)
Monday through Friday, 10:00 a.m. to 4:00 p.m. (Pacific
    time)
Web site: www.projectinform.org

The Transgender Law and Policy Institute
E-mail: info@transgenderlaw.org
Web site: www.transgenderlaw.org

WORLD (Women Organized to Respond to Life-Threatening
    Diseases)
449 15th Street
Suite 303
Oakland, CA 94612
Phone: 510-986-0340
Fax: 510-986-0341
Web site: www.womenhiv.org

Periodicals

A&U Magazine
Phone: 518-426-9010
E-mail: mailbox@aumag.org
Web site: www.aumag.org

HIV Plus
Attn: Circulation department
HIV Plus
PO Box 1253
Old Chelsea Station
New York, NY 10113
Web site: www.hivplusmag.com

HIV Positive
Circulation and Distribution Manager
Positive Health Publications, Inc.
1374 Thornborough Drive
Alpharetta, GA 30004
Phone: 678-762-0822
Fax: 678-762-0823
Web site: www.hivpositivemagazine.com

Poz Magazine
462 Seventh Avenue, 19th Floor
New York, NY 10018-7424
Web site: www.poz.com

Positively Aware
5537 North Broadway
Chicago, IL 60640-1405
Phone: 773-989-9400
Fax: 773-989-9494
Web site: www.tpan.com

Federal Government Organizations

Center for Disease Control and Prevention (CDC)
1600 Clifton Road
Atlanta, GA 30333
Phone: 800-CDC-INFO, 800-232-4636; TTY: 888-232-6348
24 hours/every day
E-mail: cdcinfo@cdc.gov
Web site: www.CDC.gov

Centers for Medicare and Medicaid Services
7500 Security Boulevard
Baltimore, MD 21244-1850
Web sites: www.medicare.gov and www.MyMedicare.gov

Health Resources and Services Administration (HRSA)
5600 Fishers Lane
Rockville, MD 20857
Phone: 888-ASK-HRSA, 888-275-4772 TTY: 877-489-4772
    (8:30 a.m. to 5:00 p.m. EST, weekdays, except Federal holidays)
Web site: www.HRSA.gov

National Institutes of Health (NIH)
9000 Rockville Pike
Bethesda, MD 20892
Phone: 301-496-4000, TTY 301-402-9612
Web site: www.NIH.gov

Office of Minority Health
Resource Center
PO Box 37337
Washington, DC, 20013-7337.
Phone: 800-444-6472 Bilingual (English/Spanish) Information
    Specialists
TDD 301-251-1432
Web site: www.Minorityhealth.hss.gov

Office of Women's Health
200 Independence Avenue, S.W. Washington, DC 20201
Phone: 800-994-9662, TDD: 888-220-5446 (Monday through
    Friday, 9:00 a.m. to 6:00 p.m. EST, closed on Federal holidays)
Web site: www.Womenshealth.gov

United States Department of Agriculture (USDA)
USDA Center for Nutrition Policy and Promotion
3101 Park Center Drive

Alexandria, VA 22302-1594
Phone: 888-779-7264, 8:00 a.m. to 3:00 p.m. EST (Monday
through Friday, closed on Federal holidays)
Web site: www.usda.gov or www.myplate.gov

Nonfederal Government Organizations

ON-LINE RESOURCES
www.AIDS.gov
www.aidsinfo.nih.gov
www.AIDSInfoNet.org
www.AIDSmeds.com

AIDS Treatment News
www.aidsnews.com
www.Avert.org

CDC National Prevention Information Network
www.cdcnpin.org
www.HIVandHepatitis.com

National Association of People of AIDS Research
http://www.oar.nih.gov
www.NAPWA.org

Women
www.thewellproject.org
www.womenchildrenhiv.org

Pharmaceutical Companies

Boehringer-Ingelheim Pharmaceuticals
900 Ridgebury Road
Ridgefield, CT 06877
Phone: 800-556-8317

Fax: 203-791-6234
Web site: www.boehringer-ingelheim.com

Bristol Myers Squibb
Corporate Headquarters
345 Park Avenue
New York, NY 10154
Phone: 800-332-2056
Web site: www.bms.com

Gilead Sciences
333 Lakeside Drive
Foster City, CA 94404
Phone: 800-445-3235
Fax: 650-578-9264
Web site: www.gilead.com

Merck
One Merck Drive
PO Box 100
Whitehouse Station, NJ 08889-0100
Phone: 908-423-1000
www.merck.com

Tibotec
1125 Trenton-Harbourton Road
Titusville, NJ 08560
Phone: 609-730-2000
Fax: 609-730-7501
Web site: www.tibotec.com

ViiV Healthcare
Five Moore Drive
Research Triangle Park, NC 27709-3398
Phone: 877-844-8872

Nutrition

The following information relates to some of the information
   discussed in Chapter 4
www.tufts.edu/med/nutrition-infection/hiv/health.html
http://sis.nlm.nih.gov/hiv/nutrition.html
http://www.cnpp.usda.gov/dietaryguidelines.htm

Bibliography

Chapter 1

http://www.cdc.gov/hiv
http://www.aids.gov
http://www.thebody.com

Chapter 2

Gifford, A., Lorig, K., Laurent, D., and Gonzales, V. (2005). *Living well with HIV and AIDS.* Boulder, CO: Bull Publishing Company.

Health Resources and Services Administration/HIV/AIDS Bureau (http://hab.hrsa.gov)

http://www.hivguidelines.org

http://www.thebody.com

Chapter 3

Gifford, A., Lorig, K., Laurent, D., and Gonzales, V. (2005). *Living well with HIV and AIDS.* Boulder, CO: Bull Publishing Company.

Guide for HIV/AIDS Clinical Care. (January, 2011). U.S. Department of Health and Human Services.

Centers for Disease Control (http://www.cdc.gov)

Office of Women's Health (http://www.womenshealth.gov)

Chapter 4

Gifford, A., Lorig, K., Laurent, D., and Gonzales, V. (2005). *Living well with HIV and AIDS.* Boulder, CO: Bull Publishing Company.

Guide for HIV/AIDS Clinical Care. (January, 2011). U.S. Department of Health and Human Services.

Nutritional Guide for Providers and Clients. (June, 2002). U.S. Department of Health and Human Services.

Centers for Disease Control (http://www.cdc.gov)

U.S. Department of Health and Human Services (http://sis.nlm.nih.gov)

U.S. Department of Agriculture (http://www.choosemyplate.gov)

http://www.aidsinfonet.org/fact_sheets/view/802

http://www.thebody.com

Chapter 5

Lohse, N., Hansen, A., Penersen, G. et al. (2007). Survival of persons with and without HIV infection in Denmark, 1995-2005. *Annals Internal Medicine*, 146:87–95.

Kitahata, J., Gange, S.J., Abraham, A.G. et al., for the NA-ACCORD Investigators. (2009). Effect of early versus deferred antiretroviral therapy for HIV on survival. *New England Journal of Medicine*, 360:1815–1826.

Panel on Antiretroviral Guidelines for Adults and Adolescents. (January 10, 2011). *Guidelines for the use of antiretroviral agents in HIV-1 infected adults and adolescents.* Department of Health and Human Services. Available at http://aidsinfo.nih.gov/contentfiles/AdultandAdolescentGL.pdf

Chapter 6

Enriquez, M. and McKinsey, D. (2011). Strategies for HIV treatment adherence success at the individual patient level. *AIDS Research and Palliative Care*, 3:45–51.

Enriquez, M., Cheng, A., McKinsey, D., and Stanford, J. (2009). Development and efficacy of an intervention to enhance readiness for adherence among adults who had previously failed HIV treatment. *AIDS Patient Care and STDs*, 23(3): 177–184.

Grimes, R.M. and Grimes, D.E. (2010). Readiness: the state of the science (or the lack thereof). *Current HIV/AIDS Reports*, 7(4):245–252.

Chapter 7

Guide for HIV/AIDS Clinical Care. (January, 2011). U.S. Department of Health and Human Services.

Mandell, G., Bennett, J., and Dolin, R. (2009). *Principles and practice of infectious diseases,* 7th ed. Philadelphia, PA: Elsevier, Inc.

Centers for Disease Control (http://www.cdc.gov)

Chapter 8

Gifford, A., Lorig, K., Laurent, D., and Gonzales, V. (2005). *Living well with HIV and AIDS*. Boulder, CO: Bull Publishing Company.

Fernadez, F. and Ruiz, P. (2006). *Psychiatric aspects of HIV/AIDS.* Philadelphia, PA: Lippincott Williams and Wilkins.

U.S. Department of Health and Human Services (http://sis.nlm.nih.gov)

http://www.hivguidelines.org

http://www.healthyminds.org/Main-Topic/HIV-AIDS.aspx

http://www.aids.gov

http://www.thebody.com

Chapter 9

http://www.aids.gov
Office of Civil Rights (http://www.hhs.gov/ocr)
http://www.hivlawandpolicy.org
http://www.lambdalegal.org

Chapter 10

Enriquez, M., Farnan, R., Cheng, A., Almeida, A., Del Valle, D., Parra, M., and Flores, G. (2008). Impact of a bilingual and bicultural care team on HIV-related health outcomes. *Journal of the Association of Nurses in AIDS Care*, 19(4):295–301.

Enriquez, M., Kelly, P.J., Witt, J., Rodriguez, L., Lopez, N., Smueles, J., Romey, T., and Sweet, D. (2010). Silence is not golden: Invisible Latinas living with HIV in the Midwest. *Journal of Immigrant and Minority Health*, 12(6):932–939.

Chapter 11

Centers for Disease Control (http://www.cdc.gov)

Chapter 12

Office of Women's Health (http://www.womenshealth.gov)
Centers for Disease Control (http://www.cdc.gov)
The Mayo Clinic (http://www.mayoclinic.com/health)

Chapter 13

Office of Women's Health (http://www.womenshealth.gov)
Centers for Disease Control (http://www.cdc.gov)
The Mayo Clinic (http://www.mayoclinic.com/health)
Enriquez, M., Lackey, N., and Witt, J. (2008). Health concerns of mature women living with HIV and AIDS in the Midwestern

United States. *Journal of the Association of Nurses in AIDS Care,* 19(1):37–46.

Chapter 14

Enriquez, M. (2009). Why don't health care workers screen all pregnant women for HIV in my community? *Journal of the Association of Nurses in AIDS Care,* 20(6):426–427.

Enriquez, M., Farnan, R., Simpson, K., Grantello, S., and Miles, M. (2007). Poverty, pregnancy & HIV. *Journal for Nurse Practitioners,* 3(10):687–693.

Office of Women's Health (http://www.womenshealth.gov)

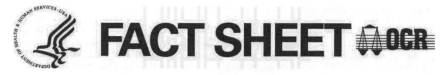

YOUR RIGHTS AS A PERSON WITH HIV INFECTION OR AIDS

The Office for Civil Rights (OCR) of the U.S. Department of Health and Human Services (HHS) enforces federal laws that prohibit discrimination by health care and human service providers. Two of these laws are Section 504 of the Rehabilitation Act of 1973 ("Section 504"), and Title II of the Americans with Disabilities Act of 1990 ("ADA").

Section 504 and the ADA protect individuals with Human Immunodeficiency Virus ("HIV") or Acquired Immune Deficiency Syndrome ("AIDS") from discrimination on the basis of their disability. The information in this Fact Sheet applies to persons who have tested positive for HIV, persons who have AIDS, and persons regarded as having HIV or AIDS.

Protections Against Discrimination

Both Section 504 and the ADA prohibit discrimination against qualified persons with HIV and other disabilities. Section 504 prohibits discrimination by health care and human service providers (called "entities") that receive Federal funds or some other types of Federal assistance. Title II of the ADA prohibits discrimination by state and local government entities even if they do not receive Federal financial assistance. Examples of entities that may be covered by Section 504 and the ADA include hospitals, clinics, social services agencies, drug treatment centers and nursing homes.

Discrimination may occur if the entity excludes a person with HIV from participating in a service, or denies them a benefit. The person living with HIV must meet the essential eligibility requirements for the benefit or service he or she is seeking. The entity may be required to make a reasonable accommodation to enable the person with HIV to participate. The ADA also protects other persons, such as family and friends, who are discriminated against because of their association with someone who has HIV.

Types of Discrimination Against Persons With HIV/AIDS

Persons with HIV infection have been denied access to social services, or denied medical treatment, or had treatment or services delayed, solely because they have HIV or AIDS. Such actions by an agency, organization, hospital, nursing home, drug treatment center, clinic, medical or dental office, or other entity, may be unlawful discrimination under either Section 504 or the ADA, or both.

Examples of practices which may be illegal discrimination are:

- *A nursing home that has space available denies admission to a person with HIV, because their staff is not trained to care for HIV-related conditions, even though the home could easily provide the necessary training.*

- *A social services agency removes a foster child from his foster home because the agency learns that one of the foster parents is a person with HIV.*

How to File a Complaint

If you believe that you have been discriminated against because of your HIV infection, you or your representative may file a complaint with OCR. The deadline for filing a complaint is 180 days from the date the discrimination occurred, unless there is good reason for delay. You may request a complaint form from OCR, or obtain one from OCR's Internet website at www.hhs.gov/ocr.

If you do not use OCR's complaint form, please write down the following information and send it to OCR:

A. Your name, address and telephone number; please sign your name. You may send a complaint for another person, providing their contact information and stating your relationship to that person, such as spouse or friend;

B. Name and address of the entity you believe discriminated against you;

C. How, why and when you believe you were discriminated against, and

D. Any other important information.

Send the complaint to the nearest OCR regional office; please see contact information below. OCR staff will review the complaint to decide if Section 504 or the ADA may cover it.

- If OCR does not have authority to investigate your complaint, we will refer it to the correct agency, if possible.

- If OCR does have authority to investigate the complaint and finds that there is discrimination, OCR will work with the entity to correct the action.

- Once you file a complaint with OCR, it is against the law for the entity to take any action against you, or any other person who provides information about the complaint to OCR. If this happens, tell OCR about it immediately.

Under Section 504 and ADA, you may also file a private lawsuit. A private attorney or your local legal aid office can tell you what the court deadlines are for filing a lawsuit.

For Further Information, Contact:
Director
Office for Civil Rights
U. S. Department of Health and Human Services
200 Independence Avenue, SW - Room 506-F
Washington, D.C. 20201

Hotlines: 1-800-368-1019 (Voice)   **1-800-537-7697 (TDD)**
E-Mail: ocrmail@hhs.gov   **Website: http://www.hhs.gov/ocr**

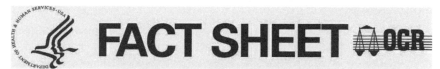

U.S. Department of Health and Human Services ● Office for Civil Rights ● Washington, D.C. 20201● (202) 619-0403

YOUR RIGHTS UNDER SECTION 504 AND
THE AMERICANS WITH DISABILITIES ACT

The Office for Civil Rights (OCR) within the U.S. Department of Health and Human Services (DHHS) is responsible for enforcing the nondiscrimination requirements of Section 504 of the Rehabilitation Act of 1973, and Title II of the Americans with Disabilities Act (ADA) of 1990, involving health care and human service providers and institutions.

What Is Prohibited Under Section 504 and the ADA?

Both Section 504 and the ADA prohibit covered entities from discriminating against persons with disabilities in the provision of benefits or services or the conduct of programs or activities on the basis of their disability. Section 504 applies to programs or activities that receive Federal financial assistance. Title II of the ADA covers all of the services, programs, and activities conducted by public entities (state and local governments, departments, agencies, etc.), including licensing.

Who Is Protected Under Section 504 and the ADA?

Section 504 and the ADA protect *qualified individuals with disabilities.* An *individual with a disability* is a person who has a physical or mental impairment that substantially limits one or more major life activities; has a record of such an impairment; or is regarded as having such an impairment. **Major life activities** means functions such as caring for one's self, performing manual tasks, walking, seeing, hearing, speaking, breathing, learning and working. Under Section 504 and the ADA, a person is a *qualified individual with a disability* if he or she meets the essential requirements for receipt of services or benefits, or participation in the programs or activities of a covered entity. The question of whether a particular condition is a disability within the meaning of Section 504 and the ADA is determined on a case-by-case basis.

What Is a "Physical or Mental Impairment?"

Physical or mental impairments include, but are not limited to: visual, speech, and hearing impairments; mental retardation, emotional illness, and specific learning disabilities; cerebral palsy; epilepsy; muscular dystrophy; multiple sclerosis; orthopedic conditions; cancer; heart disease; diabetes; and contagious and noncontagious diseases such as tuberculosis and HIV disease (whether symptomatic or asymptomatic).

Specific Requirements

Covered entities **must not**:

✗ Establish eligibility criteria for receipt of services or participation in programs or activities that screen out or tend to screen out individuals with disabilities, unless such criteria are necessary to meet the objectives of the program.

✗ Provide separate or different benefits, services, or programs to individuals with disabilities, unless it is necessary to ensure that the benefits and services are equally effective.

Covered entities **must**:

✓ Provide services and programs in the most integrated setting appropriate to the needs of qualified individuals with disabilities.

✓ Make reasonable modifications in their policies, practices, and procedures to avoid discrimination on the basis of disability, unless it would result in a fundamental alteration in their program or activity.

✓ Ensure that buildings are accessible.

✓ Provide auxiliary aids to individuals with disabilities, at no additional cost, where necessary to ensure effective communication with individuals with hearing, vision, or speech impairments. (Auxiliary aids include such services or devices as: qualified interpreters, assistive listening headsets, television captioning and decoders, telecommunications devices for the deaf [TDDs], videotext displays, readers, taped texts, brailled materials, and large print materials.)

Who May File a Complaint with OCR?

Any individual who believes that he or she or a specific individual or class of individuals has been subjected to discrimination on the basis of disability, in a health or human service program or activity conducted by a covered entity, may file a complaint with OCR. Complaints must be filed within 180 days from the date of the alleged discrimination. OCR may extend the 180-day deadline if you can show "good cause."

Include the following information in your <u>written</u> complaint, or request a Discrimination Complaint Form from an OCR Regional or Headquarters office (complaints must be signed by the complainant or an authorized representative):

- Your name, address, and telephone number.
- Name and address of the entity you believe discriminated against you.
- How, why, and when you believe you were discriminated against.
- Any other relevant information.

Send your complaint to the Regional Manager at the appropriate OCR Regional Office, or to the address located below.

Upon receipt, OCR will review the information provided. If we determine we do not have the authority to investigate your complaint, we will, if possible, refer it to an appropriate agency. Complaints alleging employment discrimination on the basis of disability against a single individual may be referred to the U. S. Equal Employment Opportunity Commission for processing.

Private individuals may also bring law suits against a public entity to enforce their rights under Section 504 and the ADA; and may receive injunctive relief, compensatory damages, and reasonable attorney's fees.

For Further Information, Contact:

Director
U.S. Department of Health and Human Services
Office for Civil Rights
200 Independence Avenue, SW - Room 506-F
Washington, D.C. 20201

Hotlines: 1-800-368-1019 (Voice)   **1-800-537-7697 (TDD)**
E-Mail: ocrmail@hhs.gov   **Website: http://www.hhs.gov/ocr**

Your Rights Under Section 504 and the Americans with Disability Act
(H-141/June 2000 – revised June 2006 - English)

Your Health Information Privacy Rights

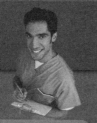

Privacy is important to all of us

You have privacy rights under a federal law that protects your health information. These rights are important for you to know. You can exercise these rights, ask questions about them, and file a complaint if you think your rights are being denied or your health information isn't being protected.

Who must follow this law?

▸ Most doctors, nurses, pharmacies, hospitals, clinics, nursing homes, and many other health care providers

▸ Health insurance companies, HMOs, most employer group health plans

▸ Certain government programs that pay for health care, such as Medicare and Medicaid

Providers and health insurers who are required to follow this law must comply with your right to...

Ask to see and get a copy of your health records

You can ask to see and get a copy of your medical record and other health information. You may not be able to get all of your information in a few special cases. For example, if your doctor decides something in your file might endanger you or someone else, the doctor may not have to give this information to you.

▸ In most cases, your copies must be given to you within 30 days, but this can be extended for another 30 days if you are given a reason.

▸ You may have to pay for the cost of copying and mailing if you request copies and mailing.

Have corrections added to your health information

You can ask to change any wrong information in your file or add information to your file if it is incomplete. For example, if you and your hospital agree that your file has the wrong result for a test, the hospital must change it. Even if the hospital believes the test result is correct, you still have the right to have your disagreement noted in your file.

▸ In most cases the file should be changed within 60 days, but the hospital can take an extra 30 days if you are given a reason.

Receive a notice that tells you how your health information is used and shared

You can learn how your health information is used and shared by your provider or health insurer. They must give you a notice that tells you how they may use and share your health information and how you can exercise your rights. In most cases, you should get this notice on your first visit to a provider or in the mail from your health insurer, and you can ask for a copy at any time.

Decide whether to give your permission before your information can be used or shared for certain purposes

In general, your health information cannot be given to your employer, used or shared for things like sales calls or advertising, or used or shared for many other purposes unless you give your permission by signing an authorization form. This authorization form must tell you who will get your information and what your information will be used for.

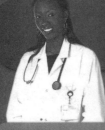

Your Health Information Privacy Rights

Providers and health insurers who are required to follow this law must comply with your right to...

Privacy is important to all of us

Other privacy rights

You may have other health information rights under your state's laws. When these laws affect how your health information can be used or shared, that should be made clear in the notice you receive.

For more information

This is a brief summary of your rights and protections under the federal health information privacy law. You can ask your provider or health insurer questions about how your health information is used or shared and about your rights. You also can learn more, including how to file a complaint with the U.S. Government, at the website at www.hhs.gov/ocr/hipaa/.

Get a report on when and why your health information was shared

Under the law, your health information may be used and shared for particular reasons, like making sure doctors give good care, making sure nursing homes are clean and safe, reporting when the flu is in your area, or making required reports to the police, such as reporting gunshot wounds. In many cases, you can ask for and get a list of who your health information has been shared with for these reasons.

▶ You can get this report for free once a year.
▶ In most cases you should get the report within 60 days, but it can take an extra 30 days if you are given a reason.

Ask to be reached somewhere other than home

You can make reasonable requests to be contacted at different places or in a different way. For example, you can have the nurse call you at your office instead of your home, or send mail to you in an envelope instead of on a postcard. If sending information to you at home might put you in danger, your health insurer must talk, call, or write to you where you ask and in the way you ask, if the request is reasonable.

Ask that your information not be shared

You can ask your provider or health insurer not to share your health information with certain people, groups, or companies. For example, if you go to a clinic, you could ask the doctor not to share your medical record with other doctors or nurses in the clinic. However, they do not have to agree to do what you ask.

File complaints

If you believe your information was used or shared in a way that is not allowed under the privacy law, or if you were not able to exercise your rights, you can file a complaint with your provider or health insurer. The privacy notice you receive from them will tell you who to talk to and how to file a complaint. You can also file a complaint with U.S. Government.

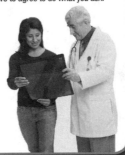

Published by:

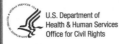

U.S. Department of
Health & Human Services
Office for Civil Rights

PAGE 2